A Practical Guide to the Eustachian Tube

John L. Dornhoffer · Rudolf Leuwer
Konrad Schwager · Sören Wenzel

A Practical Guide
to the Eustachian Tube

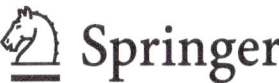

Springer

John L. Dornhoffer
Otology and Neurotology Division
University of Arkansas for Medical
Sciences
Little Rock, Arkansas
USA

Rudolf Leuwer
Otorhinolaryngology
Head and Neck Surgery
HELIOS Hospital
Krefeld
Germany

Konrad Schwager
Otorhinolaryngology
Head and Neck Surgery
Klinikum Fulda
Fulda
Germany

Sören Wenzel
Otorhinolaryngology
Head and Neck Surgery
Pinneberg
Germany

ISBN 978-3-540-78637-5   ISBN 978-3-540-78638-2   (eBook)
DOI 10.1007/978-3-540-78638-2
Springer Heidelberg New York Dordrecht London

Printed on acid-free paper

Springer is part of Springer Science+Business Media (www.springer.com)

Contents

Clinical Anatomy of the Eustachian Tube

- *Eustachian tube assessment methods*
- *Cartilage*
- *Lumen: Rüdinger's safety canal, auxiliary gap and microturbinates*
- *Muscles*
- *Ligaments*
- *Medial and lateral Ostmann's fat pad*

1.1 Introduction

Although there were very early postulations of an airway between the middle ear and the upper airway by Aristotle [40], Bartolomeo Eustachio was the first to exactly describe the auditory tube [146]. It was Valsalva who posthumously suggested naming the auditory tube after its discoverer [7]. Eustachio believed that the tube had to be open under normal conditions [155]. Also, the anatomist Duverney claimed the Eustachian tube (ET) to be permanently open, but he described the airway as bidirectional and claimed there was a second function of the tube: the clearance of fluids from the middle ear [40].

The Eustachian tube anatomy and its clinical significance have been studied using human cadaveric temporal bone specimens as well as CT and MRI studies of living subjects [191]. However, some details should still be discussed.

The Eustachian tube is divided into an osseous posterolateral and a fibrocartilaginous anteromedial portion. Whereas the osseous portion is mainly formed by the petrous part of the temporal bone, the anatomy of the flexible fibrocartilaginous portion is more complex. It is quite obvious that the fibrocartilaginous portion represents the active Eustachian tube function, but the understanding of how the surrounding elements interact remains controversial.

For example, there is a contradictory discussion about the 3D anatomy and function of the tensor veli palatini muscle [52]. Luschka [101], Rüdinger [161] and Proctor [147] called the tensor veli palatini muscle a "dilatator tubae". Dayan et al. [26] also used this term, but they noticed that the two portions of the tensor veli palatini muscle have different mechanical purposes and thus justified the use of the word "tensor". Seif and Dellon [175], on the other hand, called the tensor veli palatini muscle a "compressor tubae". Finally, Pahnke [135] and Gannon et al. [47] described both its impact upon the opening as well as closing function of the Eustachian tube.

It is one of the key merits of Joseph Toynbee to point out that the Eustachian tube is closed at rest and that it only opens for a short period when swallowing [190].

In fact, the Eustachian tube, its numerous morphologic variations [132] and its developmental changes [36] as well as its opening and closing function [70] are still difficult to understand today.

MRI is an excellent method to assess the anatomical landmarks in and around the Eustachian tube [99]. Even the opening and closing function can be demonstrated when using appropriate protocols [93]. However, not only MRI, but also low-dose sequential CT scans are suitable to assess the anatomy as well as the function of the Eustachian tube. The resolution of these scans being sufficient, the advantage of this technique is the ability to take rapid sequential scans [113].

1.2   Orientation and Length

Starting from its pharyngeal orifice, the Eustachian tube has a posterior, lateral and superior direction towards the middle ear [146]. The axis of the tube in adults is about 45° to the sagittal, frontal and horizontal planes of the skull [216]. In children the angle to the horizontal plane is significantly smaller than in adults [196]. The axis has a shallow angulation between the cartilaginous and the osseous portion of the tube, with an obtuse inferior angle. The lumen of the cartilaginous Eustachian tube forms a perpendicular gap with a minor gyration towards the pharyngeal orifice.

The total length of the Eustachian tube is variable. In adults it varies from 31 to 44 mm [146, 216]. In newborns the tubal length is about one half of the adult's [208]. The osseous part of the tube measures about one-third and the cartilaginous part two-thirds of the total length. In children, however, the relative share of the osseous part is bigger than in adults. The osseous and cartilaginous parts of the tube interlock like a seam. The average length of the tubal cartilage is 31.5 mm [135]. This cartilage extends into the roof of the osseous part [100]. That is why the borderline between the osseous and the cartilaginous part of the Eustachian tube is found between its rigid and flexible portion. Hence, the length of the tubal cartilage and the length of the cartilaginous part of the Eustachian tube are not the same. According to Zöllner [216] the distance between the pharyngeal orifice and the isthmus is 24–28 mm, but we have to take into account that there is no exact definition of the measuring points.

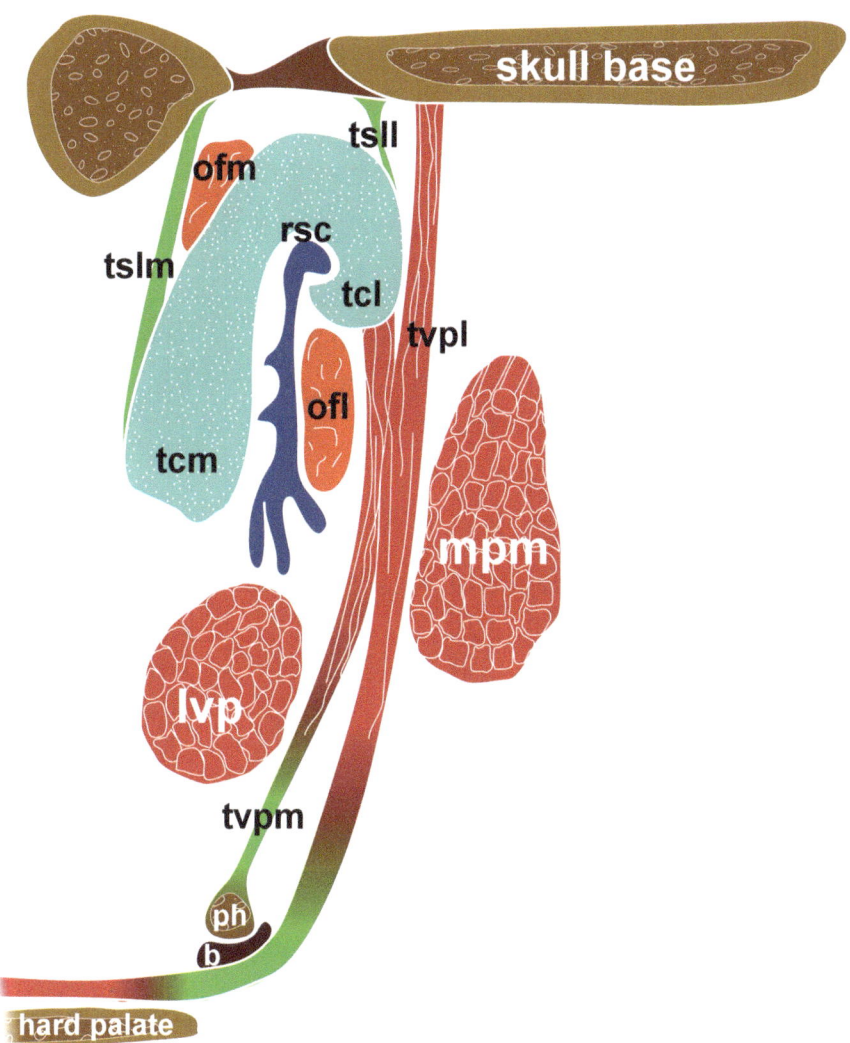

Fig. 1.1 Graphic frontal plane of the Eustachian tube. *tvp m* tensor veli palatini muscle, medial layer, *tvp l* lateral layer, *ph* pterygoid hamulus, *b* bursa, *lvp* levator veli palatini muscle, *mpm* medial pterygoid muscle, *tcm* tubal cartilage, medial lamina, *tcl* lateral lamina, *ofm* medial Ostmann's fat pad, *ofl* lateral Ostmann's fat pad, *tslm* medial tubal suspensory ligament, *tsll* lateral tubal suspensory ligament, *rsc* Rüdinger's safety canal

1.3 Compartments

Figure 1.1 is a graphic frontal plane of the Eustachian tube and shows its main compartments: the cartilage, the lumen, the ligaments, the Ostmann's fat pad and the muscles.

Fig. 1.2 Histological specimen of the Eustachian tube near the skull base. Note the minor height of the medial lamina of the tubal cartilage (*from the historical Wittmaack-collection, Hamburg University Medical School*). *lsl* lateral tubal suspensory ligament, *ll* lateral lamina of the tubal cartilage, *ml* medial lamina of the tubal cartilage, *tvp* tensor veli palatini muscle, *of* Ostmann's fat pad, *mf* mucosal folds

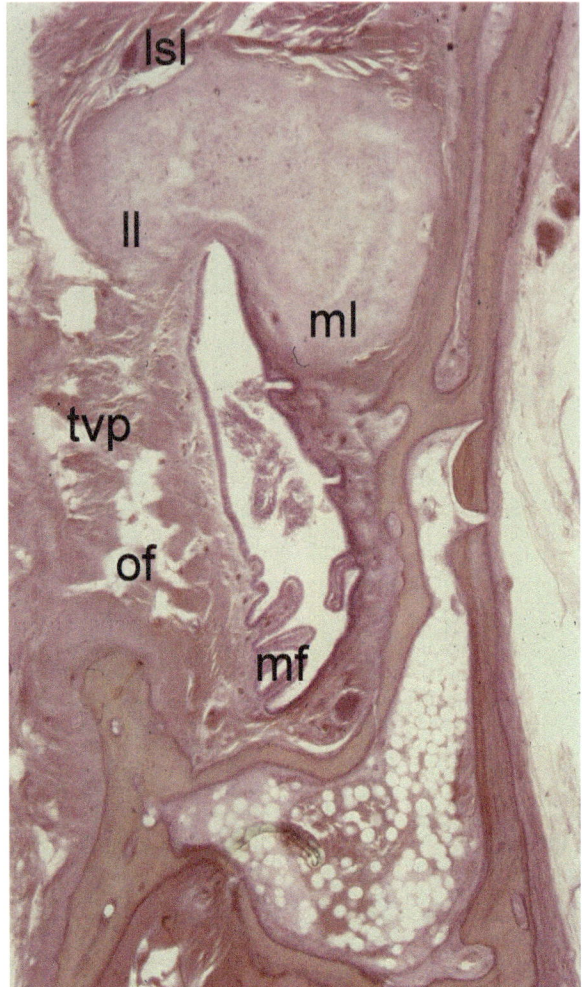

1.3.1 Cartilage

The cartilage of the Eustachian tube is one of the most important structures for understanding Eustachian tube function. Together with the tensor veli palatini muscle, it almost completely surrounds its fibrocartilaginous portion [132]. The cross section of the cartilage close to the pharyngeal orifice shows that it is "a dome-shaped structure with arms of different lengths" [12]. In other words, it forms the shape of a shepherd's crook with a bigger medial and a smaller lateral lamina [161, 216]. The mean height of the medial lamina is 5.1 mm and that of the lateral lamina 1.8 mm. The lateral lamina has a much more constant height than the medial (Fig. 1.2). The thickness of both parts is equal in the middle portion of the Eustachian tube. In comparison to the medial lamina, the lateral lamina becomes thinner towards both orifices. The transition zone between each lamina is not precisely defined [136]. Oshima et al. [132] found a wide variation of the actual shape of the cartilage using MRI studies. The physiological background of these variations still is unknown. Pahnke [136] described that in about 25 % of his specimens, the lower end of the medial lamina forms a hook around the lower portion of the Eustachian tube lumen. In some cases fragments of cartilage seem to be separated from the main cartilage. These fragments can be found on both sides of the medial lamina of the cartilage [161]. However, tracing the adjacent histological specimen shows that there is a continuous connection in most cases [5].

There is a gradual transition between the osseous and the fibrocartilaginous part of the Eustachian tube. Rüdinger [161] could show that there is a fibrocartilaginous mass connecting the bone on one hand and the hyaline cartilage on the other hand. That is why the length of the cartilage alone (31.2 mm) differs from the length of the cartilaginous part of the Eustachian tube (26 mm). Occasionally the cartilage may even reach the tympanic orifice of the tube [135].

The medial layer of the tensor veli palatini muscle is attached to the lateral lamina of the cartilage except for the anterior quarter of the fibrocartilaginous portion. The levator veli palatini muscle has a very constant relationship to the anterior part of the cartilage. However, there is no direct contact between muscle and cartilage [73].

The elasticity of the tubal cartilage is similar to that of the pinna or the nose [12]. Matsune et al. [109] examined the density of elastin in the intermediate portion between the medial and the lateral lamina of human Eustachian tube cartilage specimens. It was higher in adults. They believe that this elasticity is mandatory for reset forces after the contraction of the tensor veli palatini muscle.

1.3.2 Lumen

The lumen of the Eustachian tube is remarkable because it is not a tube. According to Rüdinger [161], the cross-sectional view through the lumen shows two different compartments:

A. The first compartment is a half-cylindrical space between the medial and the smaller lateral lamina of the tubal cartilage with a diameter of 0.4–0.5 mm, which is called *Rüdinger's safety canal* (Fig. 1.3, from [161]). This space is filled with air or with mucus. It is found in about 85 % of adult individuals [135]. Honjo et al. [70] could visualize this canal in two different X-ray examinations using contrast media. This space is likely always open [161].

B. Below the safety canal, there is a second space Rüdinger called the "auxiliary gap". This gap plays an important role in clearance and protection. Although we usually talk about the Eustachian "tube", the term "gap" helps to understand the complex Eustachian tube function.

Inside the auxiliary gap, there are longitudinal mucosal folds [161]. These folds are mainly located in the posterior, i.e. medial, wall of the gap. There are significant differences in the number of these folds in paediatric and adult

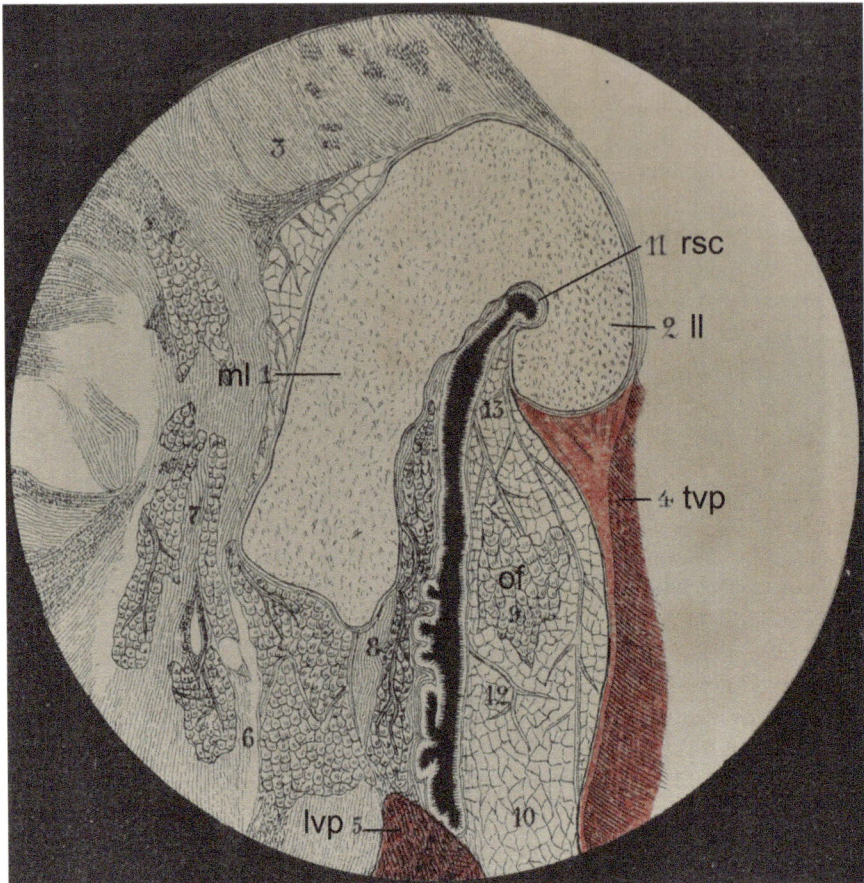

Fig. 1.3 Original illustration from the first edition of [161], showing Rüdinger's safety canal in humans. *rsc* Rüdinger's safety canal, *ll* lateral lamina of the tubal cartilage, *ml* medial lamina of the tubal cartilage, *tvp* tensor veli palatini muscle, *of* (lateral) Ostmann's fat pad, *lvp* levator veli palatini muscle

populations. Sando et al. [168] and Ozturk et al. [134] emphasize that these "microturbinates" may contribute to the clearance and protection function of the auxiliary gap.

Matsune et al. [109] could demonstrate that there is mucosa-associated lymphatic tissue within the cartilaginous portion of the Eustachian tube. Lymphatic tissue of the nasopharynx, however, does not extend into the tube [5]. The pharyngeal tonsil may reach the tubal torus and may even deform it, but this does not necessarily induce a tube malfunction [164]. On the other hand, children with recurrent otitis media with effusion may benefit from adenoidectomy due to the removal of an infectious source rather than from the removal of the adenoidal mass [138].

Between the tympanal and the pharyngeal orifice, the vertical diameter of the tube increases from a minimum of 3.5 mm in the petrous portion of the temporal bone [12] to a maximum of 6–10 mm at 6–7 mm proximally to the pharyngeal orifice [135]. The increase is not necessarily continuous. For example, close to the pharyngeal orifice, there is a local dilation of the lumen called *Kirchner's diverticulum*.

1.3.3 Ligaments

The cartilaginous part of the Eustachian tube is firmly attached posteriorly to the osseous orifice by fibrous bands [36] and to the skull base by the superior tubal ligament [147]. This ligament is also called the tubal suspensory ligament [216]. Due to a small fat pad behind the medial lamina of the cartilage, the so-called medial Ostmann's fat pad, the fibrous plate is divided into a lateral and a medial suspensory ligament. Both ligaments reach the tubal cartilage laterally and medially in a nearly tangential way. The lateral suspensory ligament passes into the tendon of the lateral layer of the tensor veli palatini muscle. On the superficial side of the tensor veli palatini muscle, there is a fascia called the *Weber–Liel* fascia. This fascia arises from the skull base and separates the tensor from the medial pterygoid muscle. We learn more about this fascia in Chap. 3. There is another fascial plate on the medial side of the tensor muscle. This facia is connected to the lateral lamina of the tubal cartilage and passes the lateral boundary of the lateral Ostmann's fat pad. The lower end of this fascia passes into the salpingopharyngeal fascia, also called *von Tröltsch* fascia. Hence, strong fasciae that connect the Eustachian tube and the pharynx encase the tensor veli palatini muscle.

1.3.4 Membranous Wall

1.3.4.1 Ostmann's Fat Pad

The non-cartilaginous inferolateral wall of the Eustachian tube is called the membranous wall. It is formed by three anatomic compartments: the tensor veli palatini muscle, the levator veli palatini muscle and the lateral Ostmann's fat pad. Rüdinger [161] called this wall "muscular wall" because the membranous wall is in fact a tendinous membrane of the tensor veli palatini muscle.

The (lateral) Ostmann's fat pad is a constant structure located between the tensor veli palatini muscle and the Eustachian tube lumen. In a cross-sectional view, it is triangular with its base located inferiorly [195]. Due to its static pressure, the fat pad helps to close the Eustachian tube. This passive closing effect can prevent the ascension of fluids and acoustic noise from the nasopharynx towards the middle ear [216] and the evacuation of the middle ear due to sniffing [105, 107], respectively.

The maximum thickness of the Ostmann's fat pad in a cross-sectional view averages 2.4 mm. This maximum is located at about 20 mm dorsolateral of the pharyngeal orifice. From this point the Ostmann's fat pad gradually decreases towards the pharyngeal orifice whereas at the same time the number of glands within the lateral wall of the Eustachian tube increases [136]. Pahnke [137] was the first to describe the impact of the fat pad upon the muscular components of the Eustachian tube. He hypothesized that the Ostmann's fat pad is a fulcrum (*hypomochlion*) transferring the pressure of the contracting tensor muscle to the lower portion of the Eustachian tube. Thus, the Ostmann's fat pad limits the opening of the Eustachian tube to its superior aspect, including Rüdinger's safety canal [195].

Ostmann's fat pad decreases in size with age [4]. This physiological decrease does not result in the development of a patulous Eustachian tube although it has been assumed that the loss of Ostmann's fat pad is the major contributor for this disorder [214].

1.3.4.2 Muscles

There are three muscles in the immediate vicinity of the Eustachian tube: the levator, the tensor veli palatini muscle and the salpingopharyngeal muscle (Fig. 1.4). The function of each muscle as well as its impact upon Eustachian tube function remains a matter of discussion [93].

1.3.4.2.1 Levator Veli Palatini Muscle

The levator veli palatini muscle originates at the lower surface of the petrous part of the temporal bone, passes the constrictor pharyngis muscle and finally spreads out into the soft palate. Its motor innervation a branch of the glossopharyngeal as well as of the vagal nerve [176]. In its pharyngeal portion, the levator veli palatini muscle only has a very shallow contact to the inferior edge of the tubal cartilage. There is obviously no direct attachment of the levator to the cartilage [73, 135]. There is only a fascial attachment to the inferior border of the medial lamina that prevents the muscle from slipping off the cartilage [16]. The levator crosses the longitudinal axis of the Eustachian tube at the so-called tubal incisure [5]. As described by Luschka [101] the levator and tensor veli palatini are antagonists. In contrast to other authors [5, 16], he called the levator a "compressor tubae". The levator probably is an accessory respiratory muscle [156]. The data of Finkelstein et al. [42], who examined patients with submucous cleft palates and velopharyngeal incompetence, suggest that the function of the levator muscle is completely restricted to the soft palate.

1.3.4.2.2 Tensor Veli Palatini Muscle

Today, the tensor veli palatini muscle is considered the essential Eustachian tube muscle [136]. The tensor originates from the sphenoid spine, the scaphoid fossa and the lateral lamina of the tubal cartilage, the posterior half of the membranous tubal wall and the salpingopharyngeal fascia [5, 16, 56]. The muscle forms an elongate inverse triangle or an "unfolded fan" ([161], Fig. 1.5), for it arises broadly from the skull base and leads around the pterygoid hamulus with a slim tendon [216]. Between the tendon of the tensor and the pterygoid hamulus, there is a small bursa. The tensor has a lateral or superficial layer originating from the skull base and a medial or deep layer arising from the lateral lamina of the tubal cartilage [147]. Both layers may be partly but not entirely separated by fatty tissue [136]. The

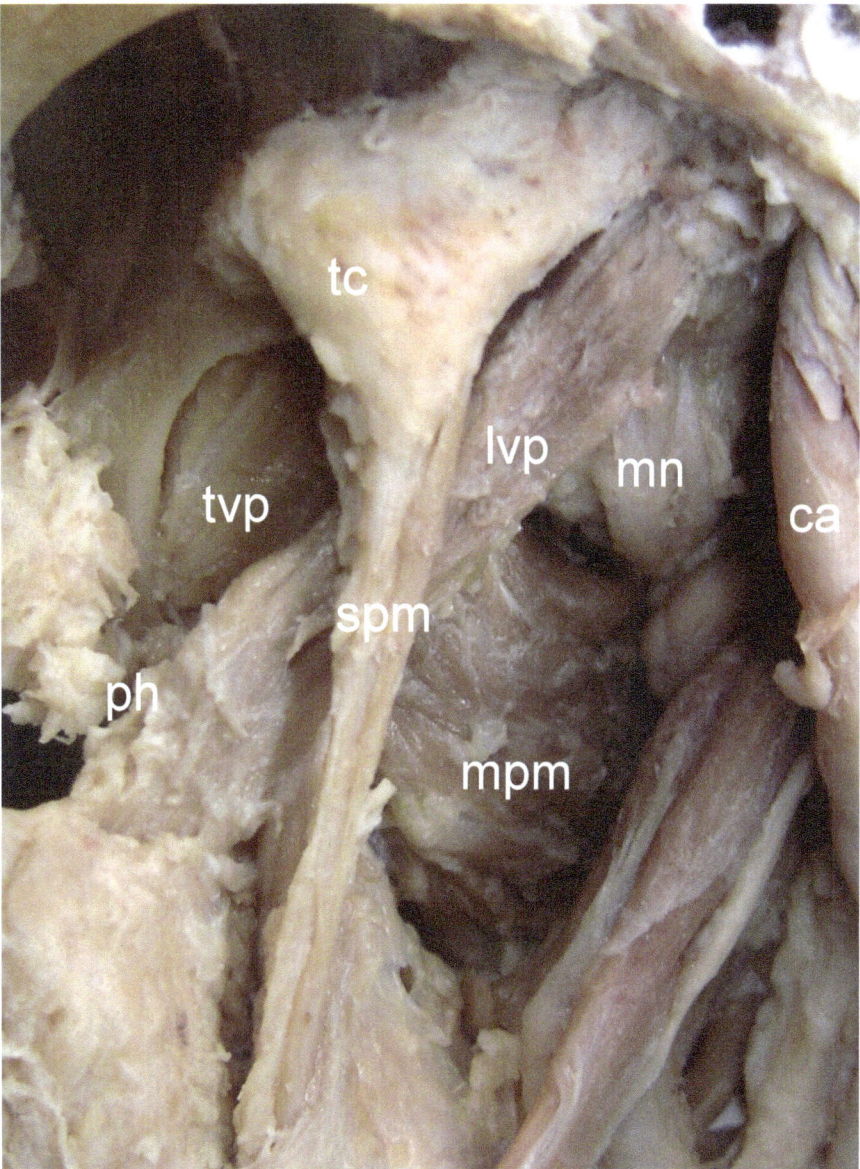

Fig. 1.4 Anatomic specimen of the Eustachian tube. *ph* pterygoid hamulus, *tvp* tensor veli palatini muscle, *spm* salpingopharyngeal muscle, *tc* tubal cartilage, *mpm* medial pterygoid muscle, *lvp* levator veli palatini muscle, *mn* mandibular nerve, *ca* carotid artery

motoric innervation of both layers depends upon a branch of the mandibular nerve [147]. According to Rüdinger [161], who only described the deep layer of the muscle, the tensor dilates the Eustachian tube by drawing the lateral lamina of the tubal cartilage away from the medial wall [56]. The force vectors of the entire tensor

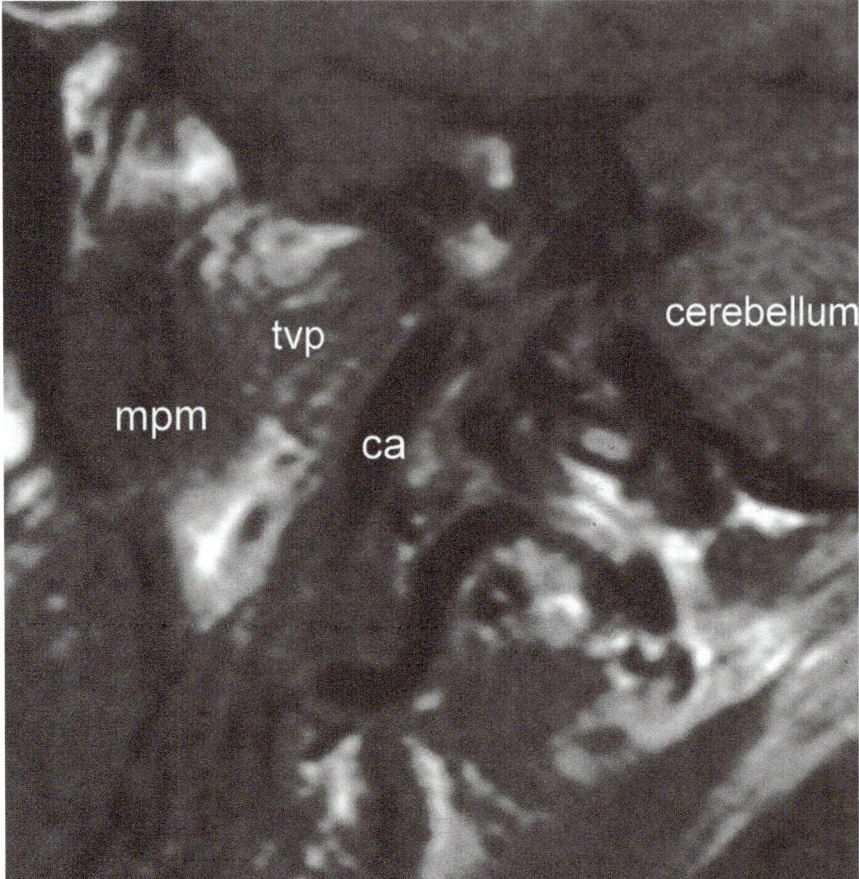

Fig. 1.5 MRI study of the tensor veli palatini muscle in an oblique sagittal plane. *mpm* medial pterygoid muscle, *tvp* tensor veli palatini muscle, *ca* carotid artery

muscle, however, are modified by Ostmann's fat pad: the concavity of the muscle pushes the fatty tissue below the lateral lamina towards the membranous part of the Eustachian tube and thus compresses its lower portion. In fact, the tensor veli palatini muscle has a dual function. It opens the cranial portion of the Eustachian tube lumen while the lower portion is compressed [135]. Thus, the tubal suspensory ligaments, the lateral lamina of the cartilage as well as Ostmann's fat pad constitute a common functional unit.

1.3.4.2.3 Salpingopharyngeal Muscle

The salpingopharyngeal muscle is a slender fibre bundle that originates from the inferior aspect of the medial lamina of the Eustachian tube cartilage. It averages 3.8 cm in length. As described by Proctor [147] its lower end inserts on the superior horn of the thyroid cartilage as well as into the posterior wall of the pharynx. Its muscle fibres are few in number and seem to lack any ability to perform physiologically [12]. Guindi and Charia [57] performed a cadaver study on the muscle. They suggested that the salpingopharyngeal muscle is adapted for sustained contraction. Between the muscle fibres, there are tendinous fibres of the pharyngotubal ligament ("Zuckerkandl"). The muscle fibres and the ligament seem to form a functional unit [216]. The thin salpingopharyngeal muscle is fixed to the farthest end of the Eustachian tube. It inserts into the longitudinal fibres of the pharynx. Hence, its inherent force seems at least to be disadvantageous. However, if we have a look at the rolling force vectors of the cartilage, this muscle gives the impression of an anchor chain keeping the pharyngeal orifice in position.

The role of the medial pterygoid muscle for the tensor action is described in Chap. 3.

1.4   Neural Control

Physiologically middle ear pressure is regulated by different mechanisms, such as gas diffusion via the middle ear mucosa, bolus-like air transport via the Eustachian tube and by tympanic membrane retraction. Middle ear corpuscles, especially in the antrum space, have been described that might facilitate pressure sensation in these areas [96]. Ceylan et al. [19] reported that tympanic glomus cells could act as chemosensory organs that are involved in the regulation of middle ear aeration. Eden and Gannon [38] hypothesized that the tensor veli palatini muscle is part of a proprioceptive feedback loop for the regulation of middle ear pressure. Songu et al. [184] examined three different groups of volunteers, of which two groups (one group with a dry perforation of the ear drum and one without) received an application of lidocaine into the middle ear and one onto the tympanic membrane. The volunteers with the intratympanic application developed a Eustachian tube dysfunction – assessed by manometric tests – whereas the others did not. They concluded that there is a neural control mechanism and that the baroreceptors in the middle ear cavity have a major impact upon this control.

Pearls

- *The Eustachian tube (ET) is closed at rest.*
- *The opening of the ET is limited to* Rüdinger's safety canal.
- *The lateral* Ostmann's fat pad *transfers the pressure of the tensor veli palatini muscle to the ET.*
- *The function of the levator veli palatini muscle is restricted to the soft palate.*
- *The tensor veli palatini muscle has a dual function: opening the cranial portion and compression of the lower portion of the ET.*
- *The salpingopharyngeal muscle is an anchor chain of the cartilaginous part of the ET.*

Physiology of the Eustachian Tube

2

- *Eustachian tube (ET) function: ventilation, drainage and protection*
- *Muscular compliance*
- *Otitis media with effusion*
- *Tympanostomy tubes*
- *Cleft lip, alveolus and palate (CLAP)*
- *ET function tests: sonotubometry and manometry according to Estève*

2.1   Eustachian Tube Function

The Eustachian tube plays an important role in middle ear function. It provides ventilation, drainage and protection of the middle ear [53, 94, 113, 203]. The Eustachian tube is open for only very short periods [36], which usually occur every few minutes around 1,000 times per 24 h [140]. Under conditions of normal function, the lumen of the membrano-cartilaginous portion of the ET is usually closed because of the pressure in the surrounding tissue [36]. That is why its key function is to protect the middle ear against reflux, organisms, sound pressure and air pressure changes in the pharynx [90, 197]. The muscular coordination of the Eustachian tube depends in part on the activity of the tensor veli palatini muscle [53, 178]. The task of the tensor veli palatini muscle is to actively open and compress the Eustachian tube at the same time. The tensor veli palatini muscle consists of two portions, a superficial and a profound portion. The superficial portion is situated between the pterygoid process and the spine of the sphenoid bone, whereas the profound portion is attached to the lateral lamina of the tubal cartilage and the pterygoid hamulus [12, 26, 52]. The mechanical impairment of the muscle may lead to a poor tubal function [94, 174]. Contraction of the tensor veli palatini muscle occurs during swallowing, yawning or movements of the mandible [203]. From its origin and innervation, it appears to be a muscle of mastication that, at the end of the embryonic period, specializes in the movements of the soft palate and the auditory tube [27].

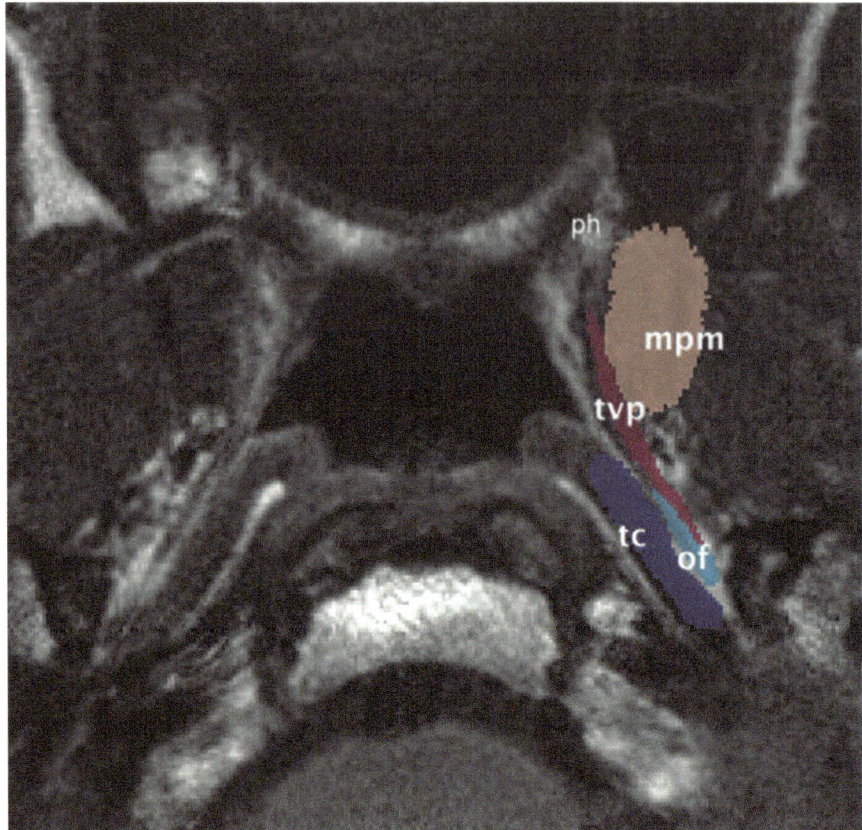

Fig. 2.1 Axial MRI study of the Eustachian tube. The critical structures are labelled. *ph* pterygoid hamulus, *mpm* medial pterygoid muscle, *tvp* tensor veli palatini muscle, *tc* tubal cartilage, *of* (lateral) Ostmann's fat pad

The muscular coordination is a complex function of the tensor veli palatini muscle: contraction of the profound portion of the tensor muscle only causes the opening of the cranial one-third of the tube (the so-called Rüdinger's safety canal) [113, 161]. At the same time, contraction of the superficial portion of the muscle compresses the Ostmann's fat pad and thus the lower two-thirds of the tube. Mucosal folds in the lower portion of the tube support a propulsion mechanism towards the nasopharynx during compression [134, 169]. Hence, the muscular coordination involves the simultaneous aeration and drainage of the middle ear by the contraction of the tensor veli palatini muscle.

To understand the mechanics of this muscle, one has to know the peculiarity of this muscle: due to its position between the skull base and the pterygoid process, with the exception of one small bursa on the lateral side of the pterygoid hamulus, it only has an isometric activity [27, 152]. That is why the tensor veli palatini muscle alone is not able to provide the muscular coordination of the Eustachian tube.

The labelling of the surrounding structures in an MRI study of the Eustachian tube (Fig. 2.1) reveals that the physiological tensor activity depends on certain

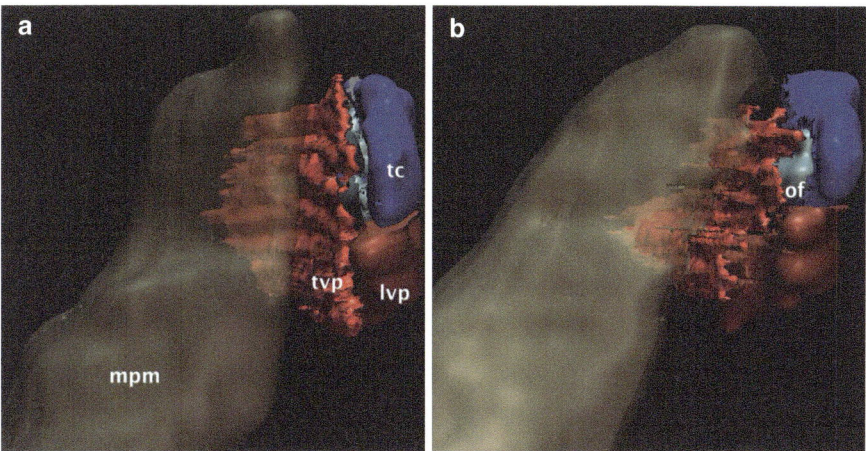

Fig. 2.2 In vivo 3D MRI model of the labelled structures from Fig. 2.1 in two different physiological states: (**a**) mouth closed (contraction of medial pterygoid muscle) and (**b**) mouth opened (relaxation). Relaxation of the medial pterygoid muscle rotates the tensor veli palatini muscle in an anterolateral direction off the lumen of the Eustachian tube. *mpm* medial pterygoid muscle, *tvp* tensor veli palatini muscle, *tc* tubal cartilage, *of* (lateral) Ostmann's fat pad

anchors that change the direction of the muscle tension, so-called hypomochlia [93]. Three hypomochlia can be identified:

1. Pterygoid hamulus [12, 52]
2. Ostmann's fat pad [136, 137]
3. Medial pterygoid muscle [93]

These hypomochlia are acting as modulators of the isometric force vectors. However, in contrast to the pterygoid hamulus and Ostmann's fat pad, the medial pterygoid muscle is mobile. Hence, its contraction and relaxation changes both the position and the tension of the tensor veli palatini muscle. This can be demonstrated by an in vivo 3D MRI model of the labelled structures from Fig. 2.1 in two different physiological states: (a) mouth closed (contraction of medial pterygoid muscle) and (b) mouth opened (relaxation) (Fig. 2.2). Relaxation of the medial pterygoid muscle rotates the tensor veli palatini muscle in an anterolateral direction off the lumen of the Eustachian tube.

The discussion about the differential role of the various auditory tube-associated muscles in tubal function remains controversial [61]. Most researchers would agree that the tensor veli palatini muscle is the primary dilator of the auditory tube [12]. Although Hecht et al. for the first time mentioned that the medial pterygoid muscle might play a role in auditory tube function, this opinion was denied by others [35]. However, comparative anatomical findings suggest that the upper portion of the medial pterygoid muscle stiffens the anterior portion of the tube [18, 47].

Figure 2.3 is a model of the main force vectors determined by the muscular coordination of the Eustachian tube. It shows the anterolateral rotation of the medial pterygoid muscle when relaxing, the pressure forces of the lateral layer of the tensor veli palatini muscle on the Ostmann's fat pad and the laterocaudal traction of the medial layer on the lateral lamina of the cartilage. Due to the position of the lateral

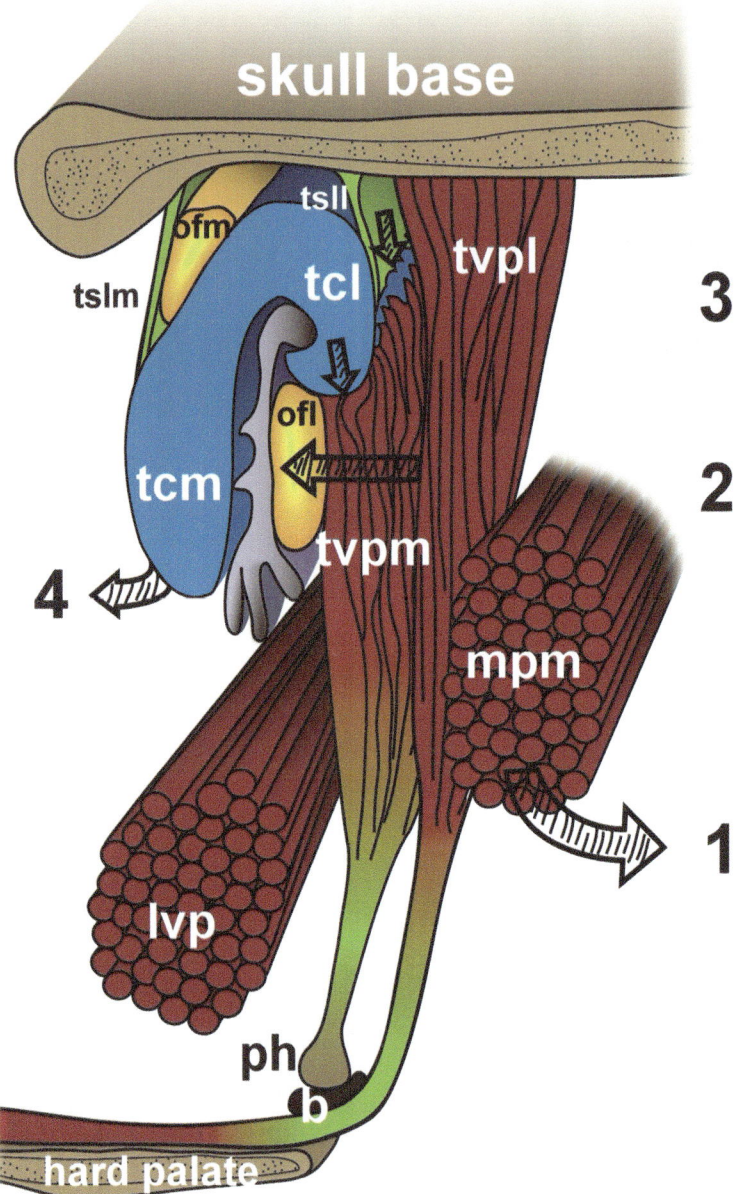

Fig. 2.3 Main force vectors determined by the muscular coordination of the Eustachian tube: (*1*)
Anterolateral rotation of the medial pterygoid muscle during relaxation; (*2*) pressure forces of the
lateral layer of the tensor veli palatini muscle on the Ostmann's fat pad; (*3*) laterocaudal traction of
the medial layer on the lateral lamina of the cartilage; (*4*) mediocranial rotation of the medial lamina
of the cartilage. *tvp m* tensor veli palatini muscle, medial layer, *tvp l* lateral layer, *ph* pterygoid
hamulus, *b* bursa, *lvp* levator veli palatini muscle, *mpm* medial pterygoid muscle, *tcm* tubal cartilage, medial lamina, *tcl* lateral lamina, *ofm* medial Ostmann's fat pad, *ofl* lateral Ostmann's fat pad,
tslm medial tubal suspensory ligament, *tsll* lateral tubal suspensory ligament (Graphical model by
Daniela Beyer, MA, Hannover University Medical School)

suspensory ligament, there probably is a mediocranial rotation of the medial lamina of the cartilage. The latter vector could indicate the role of the salpingopharyngeal muscle as an anchor chain for the cartilage.

There are typical clinical examples of an impairment of these hypomochlia. One is the loss of Ostmann's fatty tissue, which has been described as one factor for the development of a patulous Eustachian tube [137]. This topic is part of Sect. 2.3.

Another clinical example is the sequelae of hamulotomy after cleft palate repair (see below).

2.2 Epidemiology of the Diseased Eustachian Tube

2.2.1 Eustachian Tube Dysfunction in Children

Otitis media with effusion is a major paediatric healthcare issue. It is defined as a middle ear effusion without signs or symptoms of an acute infection [98]. By the age of 2, about 91 % of children will have had at least one episode of middle ear effusion [159]. The pathogenesis and duration of middle ear effusions are multifactorial. Viral upper respiratory tract infection, an immature immune system, exposure to tobacco smoke in the household and Eustachian tube dysfunction seem to play the most important roles [24, 34].

Eustachian tube dysfunction is a major problem in the young child due to the Eustachian tube's horizontal direction, its small calibre and its shortness [36]. But, when morphologically assessing the Eustachian tube alone, there is no explanation as to why some children suffer from otitis media with effusion and some do not [24, 194]. A failure of the tubal opening function has been regarded as the major problem in otitis media with effusion and retractions of the tympanic membrane. However, a tubal closing failure may contribute to the same condition [15]. In addition, the function of the Eustachian tube is impaired by the adenoids, which can mechanically obstruct the nasopharyngeal orifice of the Eustachian tube [43], provide the bacterial focus for otitis media [126, 138] or hinder velopharyngeal competence, especially with cleft lip, alveolus and palate [72, 183]. The clinical impact of each of these alternative pathophysiological mechanisms has not yet been conclusively answered.

2.2.2 Eustachian Tube Dysfunction in Cleft Palate Patients

Due to aberrant anatomy of the palate and the nasopharyngeal space [153], the cleft palate may serve as a model for understanding Eustachian tube dysfunction and its impairment.

Cleft lip, alveolus and hard and soft palate (CLAP) is one of the most frequent inborn deformities, with about 2 cases per 1,000 births [170]. The incidence of otitis media with effusion (OME) in cleft palate children is about 97 % [55]. It is important to note that the incidence of OME in children without a cleft is not much smaller. Consequently if we consider the role of cleft palate repair on Eustachian tube function [45], we should not only have a look at the early need for tympanostomy tubes [82]. Tube insertion does not necessarily have an influence on the risk of cholesteatoma, atelectasis or tympanic membrane perforations [154]. In fact it does not have an impact on Eustachian tube function at all [204]. Thus, for practical purposes, we should completely delineate otitis media with effusion in cleft children and chronic middle ear disease in cleft adults.

It is still unclear whether the extent of middle ear disease depends on the type of cleft [59]. Although the velum may obstruct the nasopharyngeal orifice of the Eustachian tube before palate repair [11], the prevalence of OME after veloplasty still remains about 70 % [158], and a very early closure does not significantly change the need for ventilation tubes [127]. According to Flores et al. [45] follow-up of patients after cleft palate repair should last at least 4–7 years in order to appreciate its effects on Eustachian tube function. In addition the neuromuscular development of the tensor veli palatini muscle generally is unfinished before the age of 7 years [59]. All surgical procedures on the growing bone and soft tissue of the midface have an impact upon the development of the facial bones [170]. Thus, it is very difficult to separate between those factors that are independent of the technique of cleft palate repair and those factors occurring by or after closure of the soft palate and which often persist during adulthood [45].

It is obvious that during veloplasty the integrity of the hamulus as well as the tensor veli palatini muscle is at risk. Thus, the muscular coordination of the Eustachian tube can be immediately impaired by surgery [9, 92]. Sheer et al. [178] used histological specimens of the peritubal space from infants with cleft palates in order to develop a finite element model of the forces involved in Eustachian tube opening. They could demonstrate two different things: the tensor veli palatini muscle force is the only direct predictor of Eustachian tube opening during muscle-assisted lumen dilations and that zero tensor veli palatini muscle force would result in Eustachian tube dysfunction. Thus, surgical division of the tensor tendon or resection of the hamulus itself, which can be simulated as a reduction in tensor force, was predicted to have negative effects on Eustachian tube function. These experimental observations were clinically confirmed by Flores et al. [45], who showed that tensor tenopexy and the abandonment of tendon transection would decrease the need for tympanostomy tubes. Our group [174] examined 15 adult cleft palate patients, 7 of whom had chronic ear disease. Eleven patients had a unilateral and four patients a bilateral CLAP. The patients were examined using ear microscopy and MRI. For different reasons ear microscopy is the only suitable method to reliably assess chronic middle ear disease [182, 211]. The patients without middle ear pathology had an intact hamulus and tensor veli palatini muscle. In all patients with chronic middle ear disease, the tensor muscle had no continuity in any of the cases as shown by MRI. In four of the latter cases, the pterygoid hamulus was absent. Thus, the mechanical impairment of the tensor and/or the pterygoid hamulus may lead to an impaired function of the tube and loss of middle ear integrity [94] (Fig. 2.4a, b).

If we consider that OME in cleft children and chronic middle ear diseases in adult patients are different entities and that the effects of cleft palate surgery upon middle ear function are visible after at least 4–7 years, it is easy to interpret a study published by Kane et al. [77]. They observed 161 children for 1 year after palato-plasty using brainstem-evoked audiometry and speech assessment. They did not perform ear microscopy. About half of the patients received hamulotomy. At the age of 2, they did not find a significant difference concerning perioperative morbidity, hearing test results and preliminary speech results in both groups. Considering the method (brainstem-evoked audiometry), the short period of observation (1 year) and the fact that most of the patients received tympanostomy tubes, this result is not amazing. Major drawbacks of many of these studies are the time frame of observation, the examination method, different kinds of palatoplasty performed and the fact that most of the children receive tympanostomy tubes [177].

The question as to whether the adenoid pad in the nasopharynx should be maintained in order to prevent postoperative velopharyngeal insufficiency still remains unanswered. According to Hubbard et al. [72], only those cases should undergo adenoidectomy in which the adenoids do not contribute to the velopharyngeal closure.

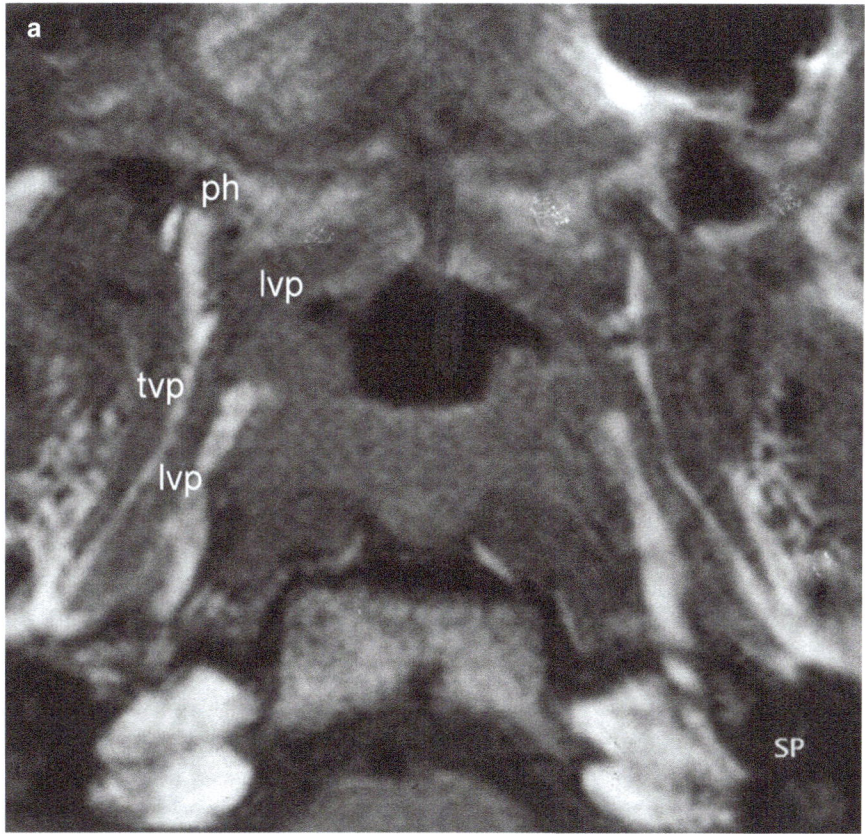

Fig. 2.4 (**a**) Axial MRI study of the Eustachian tube with a CLAP patient. Note the position of the levator veli palatini muscle after cleft palate repair. The tensor and hamulus are intact. Both middle ears are normal. *ph* pterygoid hamulus, *tvp* tensor veli palatini muscle, *lvp* levator veli palatini muscle. (**b**) Axial MRI study of the Eustachian tube with another CLAP patient. The tensor and hamulus are not intact. Both middle ears are atelectatic. *tvp* tensor veli palatini muscle, *lvp* levator veli palatini muscle

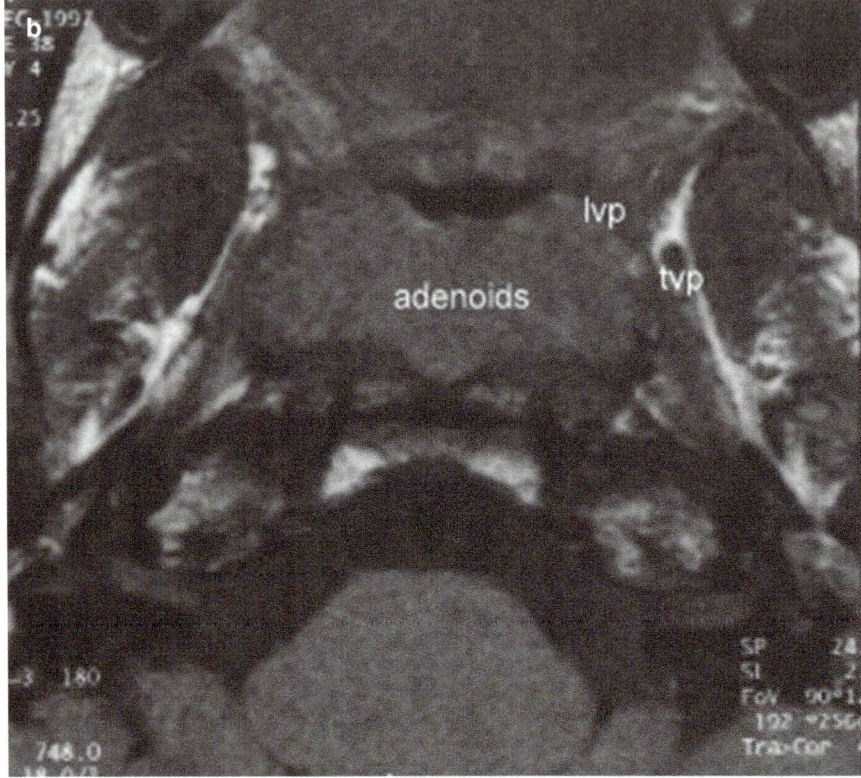

Fig. 2.4 (continued)

Because OME and its sequelae are a common problem of children with CLAP, the rational concept of an interdisciplinary follow-up with an ENT specialist is a crucial task [127]. If we reconsider the idea that OME of the cleft child and chronic middle ear disease of the cleft adult are different entities, this follow-up should include not only the young children before and immediately after cleft surgery, but also young adults. Tympanostomy tubes are a reliable tool to restore hearing with OME, but their general value for a long-term hearing improvement is controversial [98]. There are several studies in favour of a more aggressive or a more conservative use of tympanostomy tubes [82, 181 vs. 172]. The assessment of cleft palate preschool and school children by the otolaryngologist should take place at least twice a year. Bilateral OME for 6 months should be treated with tympanostomy tubes [97]. Children with CLAP have a need for long-term interdisciplinary prospective studies in order to characterize those who would benefit most from tympanostomy tubes. The focus of these studies should be identifying the treatment that will be adequate to prevent persistent hearing loss due to atelectasis or cholesteatoma.

2.3   **Eustachian Tube Function Tests**

Eustachian tube function tests should render information for the planning and especially for the prognosis of middle ear surgery. However, their relevance for tympanoplasty is highly controversial [69, 78, 207].

There are three manoeuvres described for the orienting assessment of the Eustachian tube opening: the "Toynbee" (swallowing), "Valsalva" (pressing with closed nose) and "Eppendorf" (yawning with wide open mouth).

Among the clinical function tests, there is no gold standard to assess Eustachian tube function. Most of the tests are suitable for testing the ventilation function; only a few are adequate for assessing clearance.

Tympanometry renders information about middle ear pressure and, subsequently, indirect information about Eustachian tube function. It can be influenced by adhesions, scars and an effusion [139].

In cases of drum perforations, it is possible to perform manometry of the Eustachian tube. The maximum pressures applied are about 500 daPa and −300 daPa [29]. Manometric methods measure pressure changes in the nasopharynx, in the middle ear and in the outer ear canal. The use of positive and negative pressures in the outer ear canal can assess the active and the passive opening capacity of the Eustachian tube. Swallowing when inflating or deflating the airtight outer ear canal tests the active opening; the passive opening is measured by forced inflation. In cases of an intact eardrum, it is possible to use a pressure chamber. This method has been described about 50 years ago, but its availability is very restricted [12].

At present there are two methods suitable for patients with intact eardrums without the necessity of a pressure chamber: sonotubometry [29] and manometry [129].

After more than 60 years of clinical practice, sonotubometry still has not become broadly accepted [162]. The principle of sonotubometry is to administer a sinus tone to the nose and to record this tone in the outer ear canal after tubal opening. The technique of sonotubometry has gradually improved over the years. Opening of the Eustachian tube is recorded as an increase in the intensity of the recorded sound in the outer ear canal. The focus of present evaluations is to use different kinds of sound signals. One of these sound signals – the so-called perfect sequences – has been tested by Asenov et al. [6]. Perfect sequences are broadband signals with an ideally flat spectrum. Experiments on healthy individuals demonstrated an enhanced reliability of these signals in comparison with pure tone testing. At the moment the reliability to predict middle ear ventilation is not adequate [58, 162, 203].

By using tubomanometry, as modified by Estève [39], we can register the opening of the Eustachian tube by a pressure sensor in the occluded outer ear canal. The stimulus is a calibrated gas bolus applied to the nasopharynx during swallowing [129]. The tubal opening is measured on a pressure–time diagram beginning with a pressure application to the nasopharynx. Parameters determined are the ability to actively open the Eustachian tube, as seen by the amplitude of the pressure changes in the outer ear canal, and the opening latency [29]. This promising modified tubomanometry is not a standard method for the evaluation of Eustachian tube function but has the potential to develop as such.

It is possible to study the opening mechanism of the Eustachian tube while swallowing using tube endoscopy with microfiber endoscopes less than 1 mm in diameter. The image quality, however, as well as the visualization of the lower anatomic structures of the middle ear (hypotympanon, footplate, round window) is restricted. Di Martino et al. [30] could demonstrate that the extent of the movements of the walls differed depending on the position of the endoscope within the Eustachian tube and the individual. Further studies are needed to interpret the clinical relevance of this observation.

Prasad et al. [145] examined the mucociliary clearance function of the Eustachian tube using saccharin and methylene blue. They could show that there is a good correlation between clearance time, Eustachian tube function and success of tympanoplasty. Both agents were administered through the eardrum perforations. Patients could determine the sweet taste of saccharin after its passage through the Eustachian tube; the discharge of methylene blue could be detected endoscopically. The normal passage time for saccharin was 17.5 min and for methylene blue 8.1 min. Radiographic methods, such as the measurement of the mucociliary clearance with ^{99}technetium-albumin, are not new [128].

CT and MRI can show the tissue surrounding the Eustachian tube, especially Ostmann's fat pad and the position and diameter of the muscles. To a certain extent, they can also give information about functional relationships of the muscles, but neither technique can serve as a Eustachian function test. Concerning a patulous Eustachian tube, they can even be misleading [93, 194].

Pearls

- *Key function of the ET is the protection of the middle ear against reflux, organisms, sound pressure and air pressure changes in the pharynx.*
- *The contraction of the tensor veli palatini muscle is isometric; thus, muscular coordination depends on three anchors (hypomochlia): the pterygoid hamulus, the lateral Ostmann's fat pad and the medial pterygoid muscle.*
- *Insertion of tympanostomy tubes has no impact upon ET function.*
- *OME in children with CLAP and chronic middle ear disease in adult patients are different entities.*
- *There is no reliable standard method for the assessment of ET function.*

Pathophysiology of the Eustachian Tube: The Patulous Eustachian Tube

3

- *Eustachian tube closing failure*
- *Sniffing*
- *Aetiology: loss of Ostmann's fat pad, scars and hormonal factors*
- *Therapy: medical and injection therapy and surgical methods*
- *Dynamic stabilization by physiotherapy*

3.1 Definition

The impairment of the physiological protection function of the Eustachian tube causes a distressing autophony and aural fullness, the so-called syndrome of the patulous Eustachian tube (pET) [13, 74, 130]. The pET as it is described here to a certain extent is just the "tip of the iceberg" in the general complex of Eustachian tube closing failure [108].

The Eustachian tube is closed at rest and is actively opened only under controlled conditions during respiratory rest in the nasopharynx. If the Eustachian tube is opened outside this limited range of time, there is a pathological communication between the nasopharynx and the tympanic cavity. This pathological communication causes an intermittent or constant transfer of pressure fluctuations from the pharynx towards the middle ear. Not only aural fullness and autophony, but also inner ear phenomena, such as sensorineural hearing loss and tinnitus or vertigo, and grave mental disorders are described as a result of a pET [62, 150].

The intensity and frequency of complaints vary inter- and intraindividually. In cases of rare symptoms or of low-intensity symptoms, it is enough to inform the patient of the diagnosis and of the harmlessness of the symptoms. On the other hand, there are patients who are so distressed by pET symptoms, that psychological problems arise, resulting in the inability to work or suicidal tendencies. These patients need an ENT specialist for the initiation of specific diagnostics and therapy.

J.L. Dornhoffer et al., *A Practical Guide to the Eustachian Tube*,
DOI 10.1007/978-3-540-78638-2_3, © Springer-Verlag Berlin Heidelberg 2014

The incidence of the pET is approximately 7 % [123]. Many of these patients can modify their symptoms by increasing the venous pressure of the mucosal vessels and the surrounding venous plexus of the Eustachian tube by compression of the jugular veins or by an inclined head position. In many cases "sniffing" is a useful manoeuvre to actively release the distressing symptoms. During sniffing the Eustachian tube and the middle ear are evacuated by a forced nasal inspiration, causing stiffening of the eardrum and the ossicular chain. This effect is temporary, and sniffing will be repeatedly used. The risk of a long-term sniffing habit is to produce a chronic negative middle ear pressure and the development of middle ear diseases [60, 84, 108]. On the other hand, the reduction of the intrathoracic pressure during sniffing causes a lower pressure of the cervical vein and, subsequently, of the peritubal veins and thus may even enhance the symptoms [106].

Usually the pET does not lead to a chronic middle ear inflammation because the negative pressure in the tympanic cavity is not prolonged.

3.2 Established Aetiological Factors and Therapeutic Procedures

The following factors are generally accepted as the main aetiological causes of the pET:

- Changes of the compressing tubal environment (e.g. loss of the Ostmann's fat pad after weight reduction) [150]
- Neuromuscular factors [89]
- Loss of cartilage elasticity, e.g. during the aging process [165]
- Naso- and oropharyngeal scar tissue after an operation or/and irradiation [22]
- Hormonal factors (oestrogen) [25, 141].

The reduction of the Ostmann's fat pad during intended or compulsory weight reduction [79] is considered to be one of the main factors [151] causing the symptoms of a pET. Takasaki et al. [194] observed a pET in a patient with an oropharyngeal carcinoma who developed a loss of Ostmann's fat pad during recurrence and cachexia. The autopsy showed a complete loss of the fat pad, resulting in a direct contact between the tensor veli palatini muscle and the lumen of the Eustachian tube. Using MRI Pahnke et al. [137] showed a reduction of the Ostmann's fat pad in 7 of 10 patients with the symptoms of a pET.

Modifications of the nasopharyngeal anatomy by surgical procedures, such as adenoidectomy or tonsillectomy with postoperative scarring, can also be a cause of a pET [150]. Likewise, scarring after irradiation of the cranium can also result in a closing failure of the Eustachian tube, which can be shown using tubal manometry in about 50 % of the patients [22]. After a retrospective analysis of 16 patients with a pET, Todd and Saunders [199] postulated a correlation between the frequency of chronic suppurative otitis media during childhood and the occurrence of a pET in adults. The authors maintained that this was due to a loss of turgor and elasticity of the "tubal tissue" and a change of the surface tension of the tubal mucosa due to middle ear inflammations.

The compliance of the Eustachian tube can be affected by oestrogen [3, 25]. Miller [117] documented 17 female patients in 12 years who during pregnancy developed symptoms of a pET. The largest series of patients was published by Plate et al. [141] who examined 270 pregnant women. Of these, 19 appeared to have a closing failure of the Eustachian tube but only 5 showed the clinical symptoms of a pET. The symptoms were highly correlated to the level of oestriol in the serum. Oestrogen is supposed to have an impact upon the viscosity of the intratubal mucus [44] as well as on the compliance of the tubal cartilage [141]. In addition, increased oestrogen causes increased fat metabolism leading to a reduction of the Ostmann's fat pad [188].

One neuromuscular factor is a disorder of the controlled tubal opening during respiratory rest in the nasopharynx, with a delayed closing and the consequence of a relative closing failure [89]. In addition, pathological changes of the central and peripheral nervous system must be considered, such as trauma or neurological system diseases, such as multiple sclerosis, Parkinson's disease or poliomyelitis [149].

The range of the aetiological spectrum of a pET explains the multitude of interventions suggested in order to treat the symptoms. That is why there is not an accepted standard of therapy. Neither oedema-inducing drugs [130], paratubal injections at the pharyngeal orifice [148], ventilation tubes in the ear drum [102], surgical manipulations on the tensor veli palatini muscle [206], nor a complete obstruction of the Eustachian tube [13, 31] could show more than temporary effects on the symptoms. The latter two, on the other hand, can have an impact upon the opening function of the Eustachian tube and must be regarded very critically concerning the development of chronic middle ear disease [15, 92, 167, 198].

3.3 Diagnosis

There are usually no clinical signs of a pET. In many cases the tympanic membrane and the middle ear seem normal on ear microscopy. That is why the diagnosis is confirmed by taking the exact medical history. The description of intermittent as well as permanent symptoms is as important as the past history of weight loss, pregnancy and oral contraceptives. The history should include any surgery on the tonsils and adenoids, neuromuscular diseases and, especially, temporomandibular joint disorders. Some patients complain of a pET after otitis media. If the symptoms are present on examination, they can be relieved by compression of the jugular vein. Sometimes medial and lateral movements of the tympanic membrane are visible and can be confirmed when using tympanometry. Other classical functional tests can support these findings [41, 75, 81, 124, 125]. The pressure chamber investigation does not have relevance for clinical practice due to its immense technical expenditure. MRI or CT can help confirm morphological changes of the paratubal structures but does not replace thorough clinical observation (Fig. 3.1).

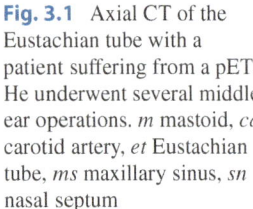

Fig. 3.1 Axial CT of the Eustachian tube with a patient suffering from a pET. He underwent several middle ear operations. *m* mastoid, *ca* carotid artery, *et* Eustachian tube, *ms* maxillary sinus, *sn* nasal septum

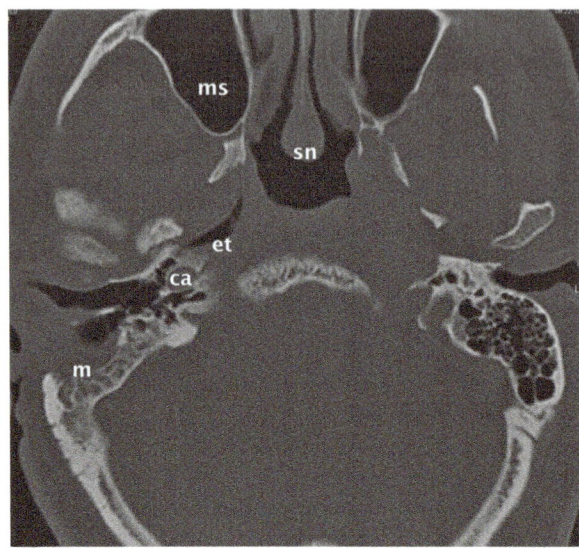

3.4   Therapy

Generally, the pET does not cause structural changes in the tympanic cavity, which thus could require a tympanoplasty. Hence, the middle ear-associated symptoms should primarily be treated on the level of the Eustachian tube. However, if a pronounced atrophy of the eardrum and a pET are present, tympanoplasty could be reasonable and should be performed using cartilage as a graft.

In cases of an oestrogen-induced pET, the cessation of hormonal contraception and other methods of birth control should be considered. Also inflammations of the upper aero-digestive tract, arterial hypotonia as well as a gastro-oesophageal reflux should be treated.

Moisturizing nasal sprays may have a supportive character in cases of a dry nasal mucosa; a sufficient therapy of the pET cannot be expected.

Oshima et al. [133] instructed their 59 patients to self-administer physiological saline solution into their noses. Their single dose was about 1 ml. The patients used the drops in a sitting position with their neck bent posteriorly. The outcome was measured after several weeks of self-therapy. They could show that this simple treatment could clinically relieve the symptoms of the pET with more than 60 % of their patients. Subsequently, they recommend this instillation treatment as an initial therapy for a pET.

Bartlett and colleagues [10] suggested loading the tympanic membrane with a putty-like substance, called Blu-Tack. Blu-Tack is a pale-blue pressure-sensitive adhesive that is produced to attach posters or sheets of paper to dry surfaces. It is a synthetic non-toxic rubber compound. They reported a temporary relief of the symptoms with 14 patients suffering from a pET.

3.4.1 Conservative Treatment

Most nonsurgical suggestions for the treatment of a pET aim at the obstruction of the pharyngeal orifice. Different authors described the local induction of a mucosal oedema by the transnasal administration of powdered boric acid, salicylic acid, trichloroacetic acid, nitric acid, phenol or silver nitrate [130, 131]. A temporary success was reported for intranasal treatment with diluted hydrochloric acid, benzyl alcohol and chlorobutanol [28], with conjugated oestrogen [31], with atropine [122] and with the oral application of potassium iodide solution [37]. The authors did not explain the mechanism of the latter medication.

An obvious consequence of the great number of patients presenting with a pronounced loss of weight within a short period of time is to suggest a "therapeutic" gain of weight first. Yet Pahnke et al. [137] could not show a positive effect after a significant increase of body weight in seven affected patients. They explained this observation by the anatomical structure of the Ostmann's fat pad: the Ostmann's fat pad is separated by strong connective tissue connecting the medial fascia of the tensor muscle and the membranous lateral Eustachian tube wall (paries membranaceus) [111, 216]. During the loss of weight, the fat and the connective tissue are affected and shrink. This process to a certain point seems to be irreversible, preventing the Ostmann's fatty tissue from regrowing once the body weight has recovered [137].

3.4.2 Injection Therapy

A therapy frequently suggested is the augmentation of the nasopharyngeal orifice of the Eustachian tube. The success rate of the augmentation therapy depends on the long-term stability rather than the quantity of the injected substance. Pulec [148] used polytetrafluoroethylene paste (Teflon®). He injected this substance into the anterior–inferior margin of the nasopharyngeal Eustachian tube orifice and observed an improvement of the pET symptoms in 73 % (19 of 26 patients) within a 3-year follow-up. According to the author, the tissue compatibility of Teflon® is good. Officially, injection of Teflon® paste anterior to the mouth of the Eustachian tube has been stopped by the manufacturer of the paste because of serious complications caused by the Teflon paste being accidentally injected into the internal carotid artery [130]. Figure 3.2 shows an MRI of a young adult German patient treated by Pulec himself in the 1990s.

Other materials have been used for augmentation and/or obstruction, such as autologous fat, collagen and even silicone. Surprisingly there are no long-term results published. Kong et al. [85] injected paste-like minced autologous tragal cartilage submucosally into the pharyngeal orifice of the Eustachian tubes of two

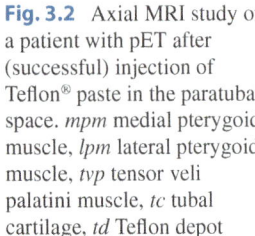

Fig. 3.2 Axial MRI study of a patient with pET after (successful) injection of Teflon® paste in the paratubal space. *mpm* medial pterygoid muscle, *lpm* lateral pterygoid muscle, *tvp* tensor veli palatini muscle, *tc* tubal cartilage, *td* Teflon depot

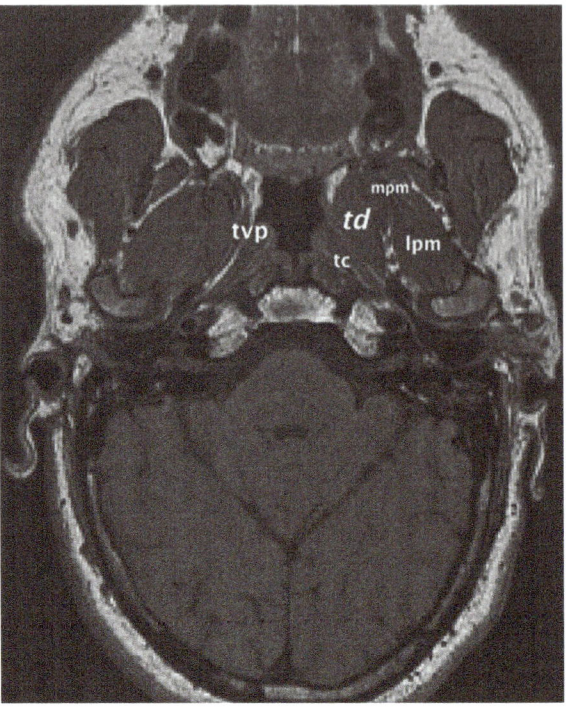

patients. Both patients remained free of symptoms for 18 and 24 months, respectively, after the procedure.

3.4.3 Surgical Therapy

The insertion of grommets into the tympanic membrane is the most frequently suggested procedure for pET [102]. The success rates are up to 50 % or higher [21, 150]. Seventy percent of these patients had breath-synchronous, tympanometric eardrum movements preoperatively. The insertion of grommets has no significant effect upon the annoying symptom of autophony. The tympanic ventilation shunt is only able to absorb the pressure changes in the tympanic cavity, which are due to swallowing and breathing. The transtubal sound transmission caused by the impaired protection function is not influenced. The uncertain and incomplete effect of grommets is additionally restricted by local side effects of the tympanostomy tubes, such as otorrhea.

Virtanen [205] suggested increasing the paratubal pressure by ligature of the internal jugular vein. Unfortunately, there are no published data on the long-term effect of this therapy. Due to the adaptability of the venous drainage, the intended increase of the paratubal pressure is temporary.

Surgical obstruction of the Eustachian tube can be performed in the nasopharyngeal or the tympanic orifice. By means of a urologic diathermy probe, Robinson and Hazell [157] could achieve a complete or partial removal of pET complaints in 9 of 13 patients. Data concerning the long-term effect (more than 3 months) are missing in the publications.

Poe [143] demonstrated a method of surgical augmentation of the nasopharyngeal orifice using autologous cartilage, an alloderm implant or calcium hydroxyapatite. He used a transnasal/transoral approach and inserted the graft under endoscopic control anterolateral to the tubal lumen. His success rates (six patients satisfied, eight patients dissatisfied) and the absence of surgical and physiological complications make it reasonable to think about a modification of this interesting technique (see below).

Yanez et al. [213] recently reported a laser-assisted curvature inversion technique of the medial and lateral lamina of the Eustachian tube cartilage. A Potassium-titanyl phosphate laser is used as a cutting tool. It is applied transorally and transnasally, respectively, using a fibre-optic tool. A cross-hatching cutting technique alters the tension of the cartilage of the pharyngeal orifice. The authors treated 11 patients and, according to their publication, they achieved a complete long-term relief of symptoms in more than 70 % of the cases.

In cases of a persistent pET after conservative therapy the authors use septal cartilage for the augmentation of the nasopharyngeal orifice. Harvested nasal septum cartilage splints measuring about 2.5×1 cm are implanted between the tensor veli palatini muscle and the Eustachian tube under full anaesthesia (Fig. 3.3a, b). For implantation a transpalatinal approach is used, which is controlled by nasal endoscopy. A navigation system can help to avoid misplacement (Fig. 3.4). Once the bed for the cartilage is formed by a scissor, the splint is pushed upward as far as possible (Fig. 3.5). Due to the good results of the physiotherapy, only seven patients have been treated using this augmentation method. One patient had no effect of the treatment between 6 and 12 months after surgery, two patients described a moderate relief, and four patients a marked relief of their symptoms. There were no surgery-associated septal or middle ear complications in this group; no patient reported sensations of a pharyngeal foreign body.

There are a lot of advantages of this method:

- Nasal septum cartilage is a stable material that is easy to harvest.
- The direct transpalatinal implantation approach can be easily controlled by telescope.
- The tensor veli palatini muscle is a safe landmark for placement of the cartilage.
- The procedure is reversible.

Doherty and Slattery [31] could eliminate autophony and aural fullness successfully in two cases by cauterization and autologous fat graft plugging of the Eustachian tube at its nasopharyngeal orifice, in conjunction with myringotomy and ventilation tube placement.

Fig. 3.3 (a) Transpalatinal paratubal implantation of septal cartilage. The testing probe is in the lumen of the Eustachian tube. *SN* nasal septum, *Z* tongue, *C* cartilage, *T* tensor veli palatini muscle, *L* levator veli palatini muscle, *TA* tubal cartilage. (b) Septal cartilage in final position. *SN* nasal septum, *C* cartilage, *L* levator veli palatini muscle, *TA* tubal cartilage, *WG* soft palate

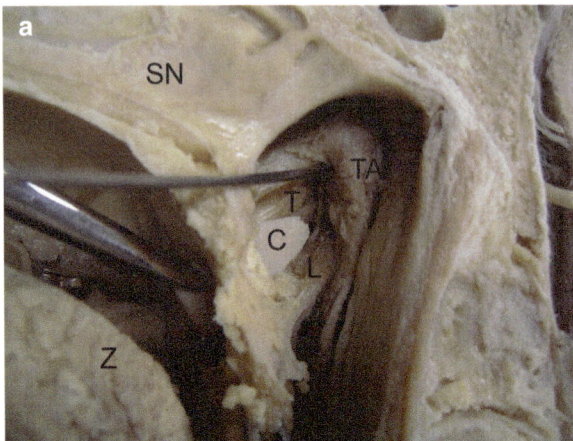

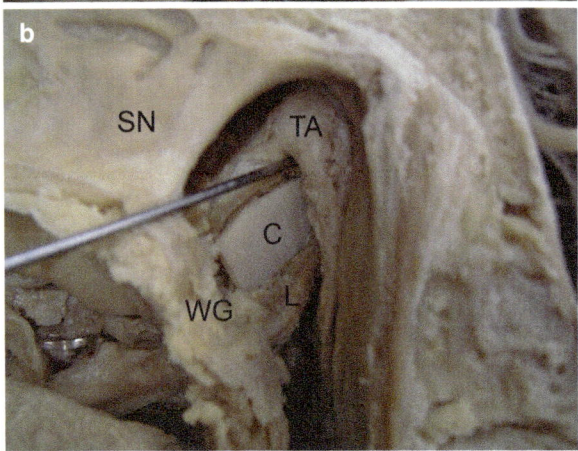

The transtympanal obstruction of the Eustachian tube was demonstrated by Bluestone and Cantekin [13] and by Dyer and McElveen [37]. They inserted a soft catheter into the tympanal orifice and fixed it with bone wax. These patients also received tympanostomy tubes for ventilation. The advantage of this method is its reversibility. Unfortunately, exact numbers of patients successfully treated are unknown.

Another technical approach is to impair the opening force of the tensor veli palatini muscle, either by resection or by toxic inhibition [120, 187, 206]. Stroud et al. [187] cut off the tensor's tendon in 10 patients with pET, with a reported success rate of 90 % (9 of 10 patients). Virtanen and Palva [206] extended the concept by the fracture or resection of the pterygoid hamulus. According to the authors, 9 of 13 patients remained without pET complaints up to 60 months. Despite the high success rates and the small rate of surgery-related complications, both procedures cannot be generally accepted in the therapy of the pET. Factures of the hamulus and surgical manipulations at the tensor veli palatini muscle are known as the

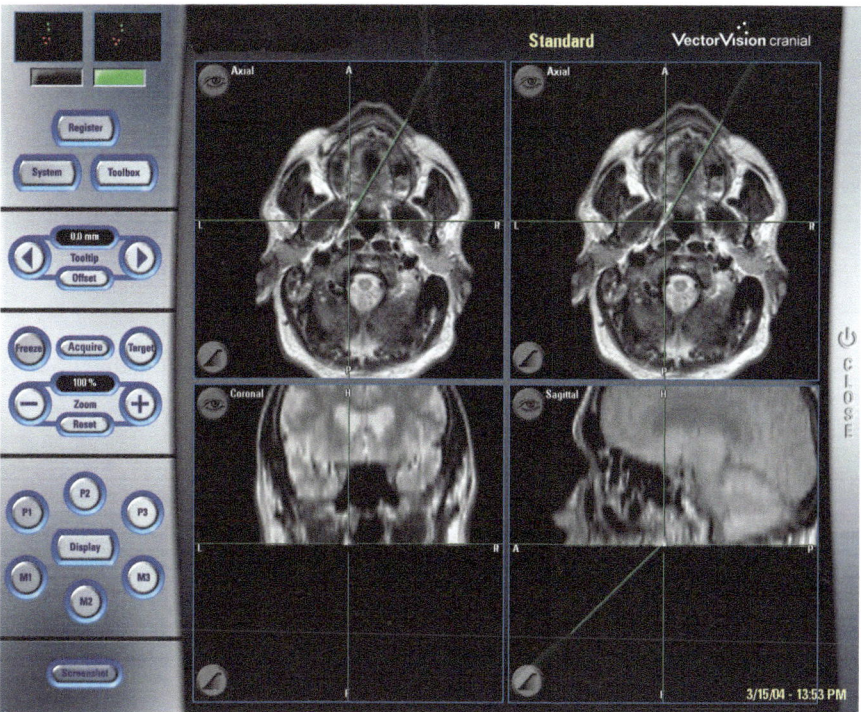

Fig. 3.4 Control of the position of the septal cartilage using 3D-MRI-navigation

Fig. 3.5 Intraoperative situation: transpalatinal approach and velotraction for endoscopic control of the nasopharynx

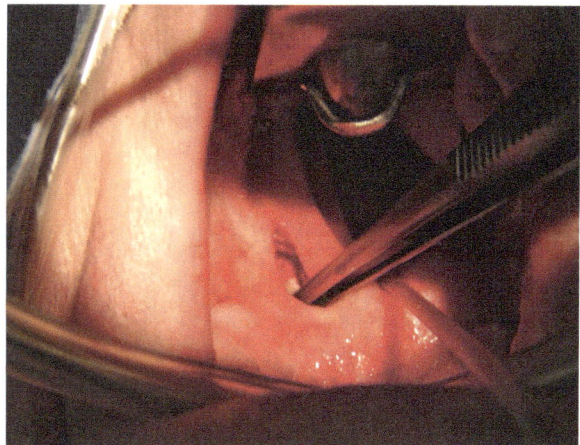

substantial causes of chronic middle ear inflammations after cleft palate closure [14, 91, 158, 181]. The tensor not only opens the Eustachian tube, but it also is the physiological basis for active drainage of the middle ear [169]. A passive Eustachian tube without active muscular coordination should be absolutely avoided.

3.4.4   The "Dynamic Stabilization"

Despite the multitude of recommendations for the therapy of a pET, there still is no standard approach for these patients. All the studies published on the topic deal with a small number of patients. In addition, there is more than one pathophysiological mechanism responsible for the individual pET. Moreover, many of the components of the Eustachian tube playing a role in pET, such as the ingredients of the mucus, remain unknown. On the other hand, due to the differential specificity of the pathology, many cases of pET remain undetected. Many of the procedures described above are accompanied by their own Eustachian tube pathology. That is why it is justified to look for a completely non-invasive approach for correcting the pET. The aim of this approach should be to reduce the symptoms of the pET and to keep the intrinsic Eustachian tube function.

3.4.4.1   Morphological Background

The tensor veli palatini opens the Eustachian tube for ventilation and provides active drainage of the middle ear at the same time. Its function depends on the medial pterygoid muscle as an active, elastic and movable modulator of the muscular force vector of the tensor, influencing the compliance of the Eustachian tube. The diameter of the medial pterygoid muscle crossing the tensor veli palatini muscle exceeds the diameter of the latter by far. Contraction of the medial pterygoid muscle provides a posteromedial movement of the tensor veli palatini muscle towards the Eustachian tube, increasing the tubal opening pressure. Relaxation of the medial pterygoid muscle results in an anterolateral movement of the tensor veli palatini muscle and a simultaneous decrease of the opening pressure [93, 94]. The mandibular branch of the trigeminal nerve innervates both muscles. The tensor veli palatini nerve branches from the medial pterygoid nerve [1, 166]. The Weber–Liel fascia separates both the medial pterygoid and the tensor veli palatini muscles (Fig. 3.6a, b). On both margins of this fascia, there are netlike fibromuscular interconnections between the medial pterygoid and the tensor veli palatini muscles. These interconnections could explain how the Eustachian tube can be opened by mandibular opening alone [17, 104]. This close anatomical correlation underlines the common phylogenetic task of both of the muscles [32].

In a series of 47 patients with the clinical symptoms of a pET, MR tomographies of the Eustachian tube region were performed. With regard to the medial pterygoid muscle, the results were non-uniform. Whereas the morphologic aspect of the Eustachian tube and of the surrounding tissue was normal in 26 of the patients, 11 had a hypotrophy of the medial pterygoid muscle and 10 had a hypotrophy of Ostmann's fat pad. Seven had both.

The active role of the medial pterygoid muscle is the basis for a completely physiotherapeutic approach [210] when treating a pET.

The aim of the concept of "dynamic stabilization" is to activate the third hypomochlion of the tensor veli palatini muscle, the medial pterygoid muscle and the paratubal muscles.

Fig. 3.6 (**a**) Anatomic specimen with crossing of the medial pterygoid muscle and the tensor veli palatini muscle after removal of the medial lamina of the pterygoid process and of the levator veli palatini muscle showing the margins of the Weber–Liel fascia. *SB* skull base, *TA* Eustachian tube (cartilage), *L* levator veli palatini muscle, *M* medial pterygoid muscle, *Nm* mandibular nerve, *Pp* margin of the medial lamina of the pterygoid process, *T* tensor veli palatini muscle, *arrow* pterygoid hamulus. (**b**) Anatomic specimen with the medial pterygoid muscle after cranialization of the tensor veli palatini muscle showing the Weber–Liel fascia. *tvp* tensor veli palatini muscle, *fi* fibromuscular interconnections, *mn* mandibular nerve, *wlf* Weber–Liel fascia

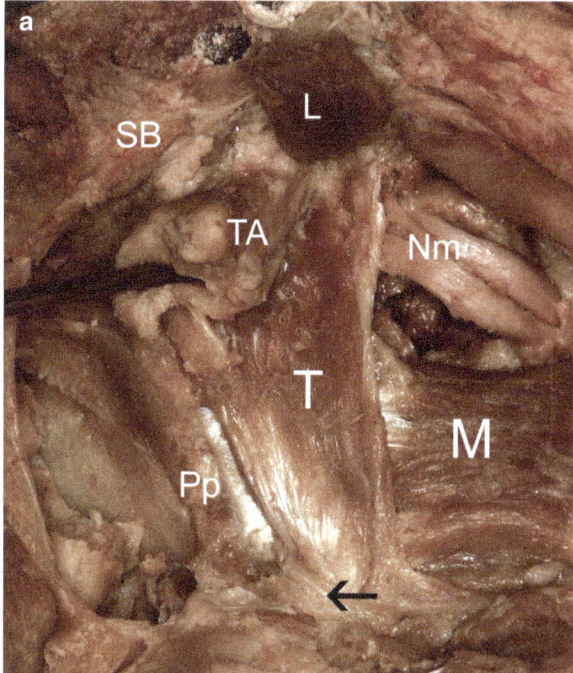

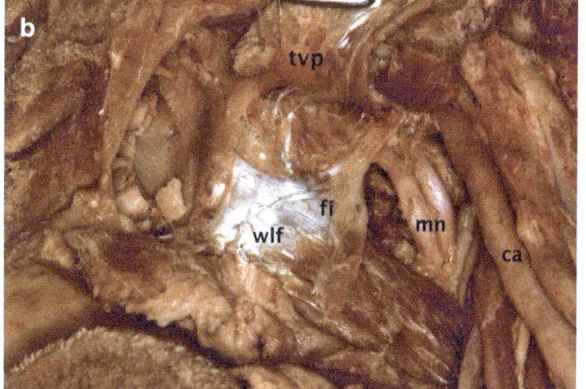

3.4.4.2 Specific Examinations

If the patient suffers from symptoms of a pET that require intervention, the following additional examinations should be performed:

1. An MRI of the Eustachian tube region (Fig. 3.7a–c)
2. The functional analysis of the masticatory muscles and of the temporomandibular joint by a specialized dentist
3. The evaluation of the musculoskeletal system of the craniocervical region by a physiotherapist (Fig. 3.8a–f)

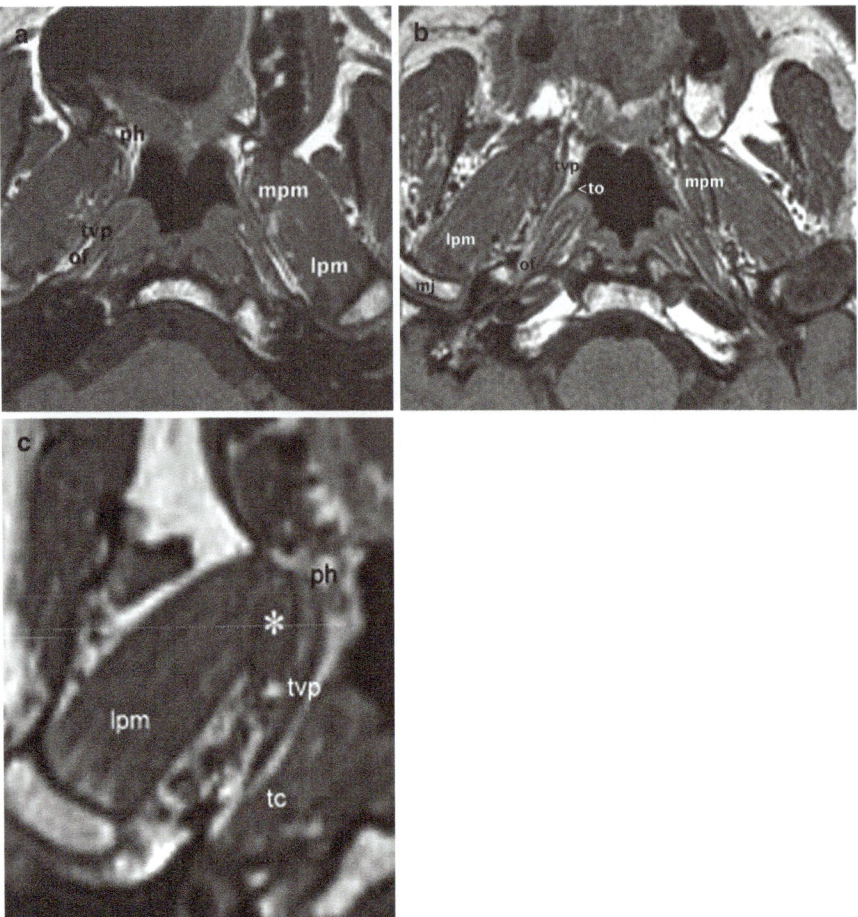

Fig. 3.7 (**a**) Axial MRI study of a healthy subject. Note the club shape of the Ostmann's fat pad on both sides and the size of the medial and lateral pterygoid muscle. *ph* pterygoid hamulus, mpm: medial pterygoid muscle, *lpm* lateral pterygoid muscle, *tvp* tensor veli palatini muscle, *of* Ostmann's fat pad. (**b**) Axial MRI study of a patient complaining of a pET. Note the thin signal of the Ostmann's fat pad. The patient is able to actively open the right Eustachian tube and to keep it opened for the entire examination. However, this ability does not prove the clinical syndrome! *tvp* tensor veli palatini muscle, *mpm* medial pterygoid muscle, *lpm* lateral pterygoid muscle, *of* Ostmann's fat pad, *mj* mandibular joint, *to* pharyngeal tubal orifice (*With kind permission of Prof. Dr. Jens Fiehler, MD, Chairman Dept. of Neuroradiology, University of Hamburg Medical School*). (**c**) Axial MRI study of a patient complaining of a patulous Eustachian tube. Note the hypotrophy of the medial pterygoid muscle (*) and the straight course of the tensor veli palatini muscle. *lpm* lateral pterygoid muscle, *tc* tubal cartilage, *tvp* tensor veli palatini muscle, *ph* pterygoid hamulus

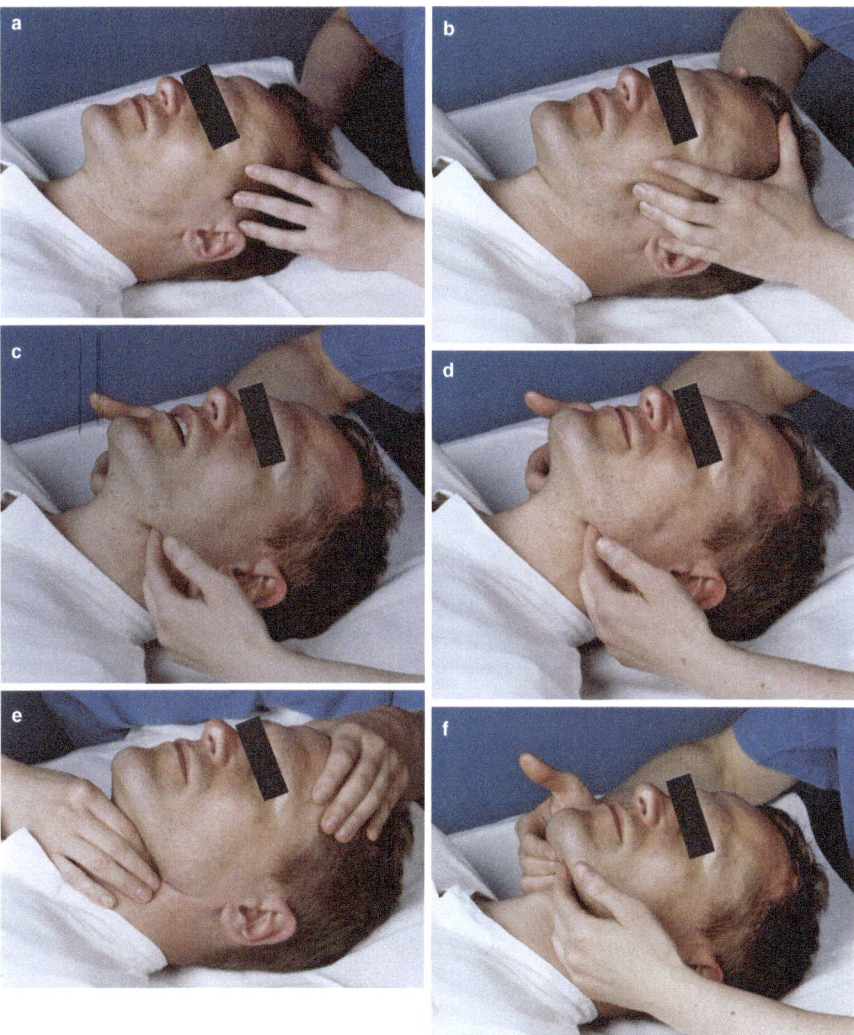

Fig. 3.8 (a–f) Assessment of the masticatory muscles by the physiotherapist. (**a**)Temporal muscles. (**b**) Masseter muscles. (**c**) Relaxed medial pterygoid muscles. (**d**) Contracted medial pterygoid muscles. (**e**) Geniohyoid muscles. (**f**) Mylohyoid muscles

In addition to an examination of the teeth and parodontium, the dental analysis includes the examination of the masticatory and cervical muscles and of the temporomandibular joints. The aim is to differentiate between arthrogenic, myogenic or combined disturbances [173]. The dental evaluation also examines the occlusion, the mobility of the mandible with maximum mouth opening and maximum protrusion, laterotrusion and retrusion, the observation of noise and pain in the temporomandibular joints, active and passive muscle characteristics such as thickness, force and inhomogeneities (masseter, anterior/medial/posterior temporal,

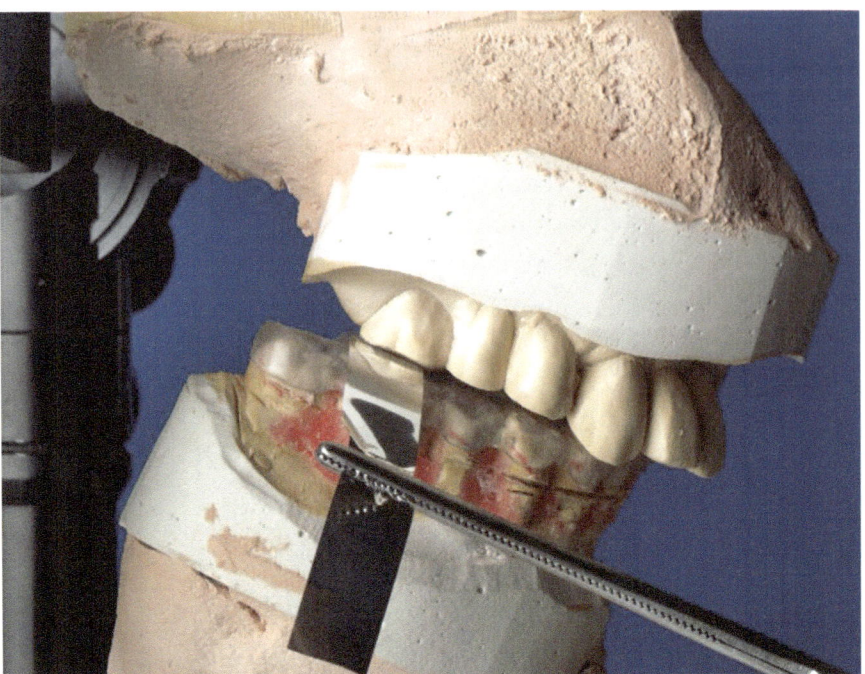

Fig. 3.9 Adjustment of individual occlusal splints

sternocleidomastoideus, trapezoid, suprahyoid, digastric and medial and lateral pterygoid muscles) and the identification of parafunctional findings (cheek changes, abrasions, tooth loosening, etc.).

The physical examination by the dentist is needed for the planning of physiotherapy and for the support of the physiotherapy by individual splints (Fig. 3.9). One goal of such an occlusal splint is to strengthen the ipsilateral medial pterygoid muscle by contralateral relief.

3.4.4.3 Eustachian Tube-Specific Physiotherapy

The physiotherapist must consider the cervical and masticatory muscles, including the floor of the mouth, as a biomechanical unit. All these muscles are connected like a chain, either by direct contact or by common structures for insertion, such as the hyoid bone and the palatine aponeurosis [118, 160]. Special interest is given to the basic tension and to the function of the cervical and masticatory muscles by inspection and by palpation.

Typical findings are:

- Loss of the cervical spine lordosis with hypertension and shortening of the ventral musculature (in particular hyoid bone and mylohyoid muscle)
- Cervical spine hyperlordosis with hypertension and shortening of the masticatory muscles with a decrease of the vertical and horizontal motion amplitude and a pathological opening of the mouth (Fig. 3.10a, b)

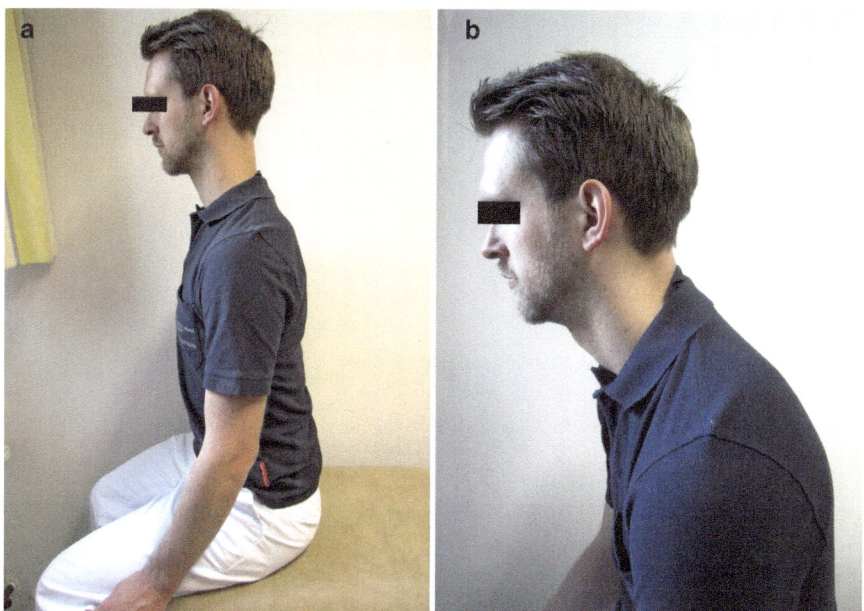

Fig. 3.10 (**a**) Physiological posture of the cervical spine. (**b**) Unphysiological posture of the cervical spine (*With kind permission of Christiane Keller, University of Düsseldorf Medical School*)

Thirty-four of the 47 patients examined with a pET (three-quarters) showed an early protrusion of the mandible during mouth opening; 22 had lateral shifts from the mediosagittal plane together with morphologic and functional differences of the masticatory muscles of each side. A shortening of the occlusal muscles, like the medial pterygoid muscle, caused lateral deviations to the symptomatic pET side. This shortening has an impact on the function of the third hypomochlion of the Eustachian tube and thus the opening pressure of the tube.

According to the individual findings, a training programme is prepared for the patient. The main goal is the dynamic stabilization of hypo- or hyperfunctional craniomandibular and cervical muscles as well as of the temporomandibular joints.

- A hyperlordosis of the cervical spinal column with abnormal forward neck posture ("screen posture") is treated by active stretching of the hypertonic neck muscles and a relaxation of the ventral cervical and infra- and suprahyoid muscles (Fig. 3.11). This includes the development of a physiological cervical and lumbar lordosis as well as a thoracic kyphosis.
- The straight cervical spine ("reversed physiological curvature") is treated by an active stretching of the ventral cervical and hyoid muscles (Fig. 3.12). In a prone position, an additional strengthening of the nuchal and an additional relaxation of the hypertonic ventral cervical and hyoidal musculature can be obtained. A physiotherapeutic correction of the spinal column and the body position is likewise accomplished.

Fig. 3.11 Active stretching of the hypertonic neck muscles

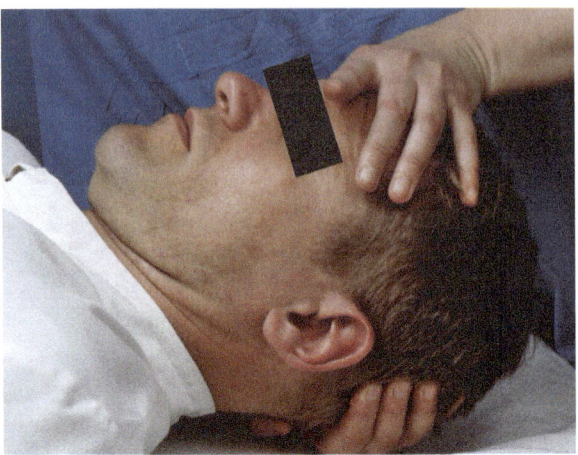

Fig. 3.12 Active stretching of the ventral cervical and hyoid muscles

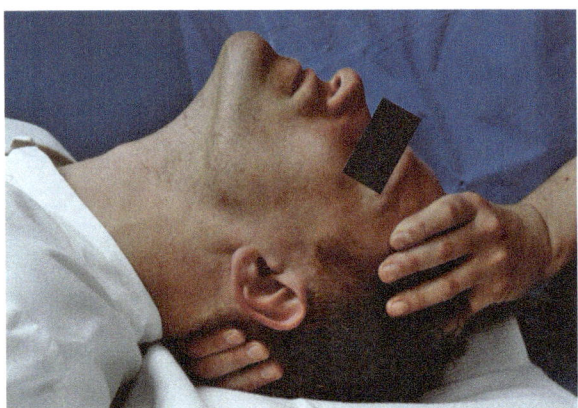

- In cases of hypertonic muscles of the floor of the mouth and an elevation of the hyoid bone, which are usually associated with a straight cervical spine, the so-called yawning respiration is exercised with a closed mouth (Fig. 3.13). This causes an active muscular stretching of the mylohyoid muscle as well as a depression of the base of the tongue and the hyoid bone.
- Failure to breath through the nose, with lowered activity of the palatine muscles but without substantial anatomical nasal obstruction (e.g. septal deviation), is addressed, and the patient is instructed to use nasal respiration. The conscious maintenance of physiological conditions in the oral cavity and in the oropharynx is also addressed. This includes the so-called soft tissue closure by loosely closing the lips, leaving a small distance between the teeth in the occlusal plane and the tongue contacting loosely the front two-thirds of the hard palate. The tongue base should not have a substantial basic tension or elevation in this position.
- Laterotrusions ("shifts"), early protrusions and muscular imbalances of the opening of the mouth are treated by the dynamic stabilization of the mandible. The

Fig. 3.13 Active muscular stretching of the mylohyoid muscle as well as a depression of the base of the tongue and the hyoid bone

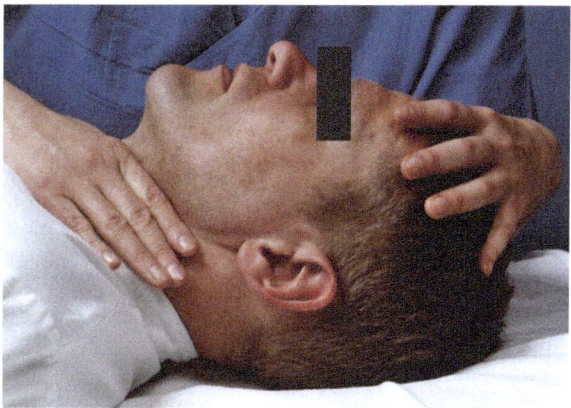

jaw depressions to a maximum of 50 mm as well as the laterotrusion up to 12 mm for practising force equilibrium are exercised without or against resistance, respectively (Fig. 3.14a–c). Patients with pathologically early protrusions of the mandible are instructed to avoid this habit consciously and trained with appropriate exercises.

- In cases of a dystonic base of the tongue, the tongue is mobilized with and without resistance (e.g. mouth spatula pressure) (Fig. 3.15). While fixing the neighbouring structures, such as the mandible, antidromic movements of the tongue and head are made. The physiotherapeutic mobilization of the tongue and base of tongue muscles always includes a mobilization of dependent hyoid bone.

In practice, the first series consists of six physiotherapeutic training units. If the symptoms of the pET persist, a second one follows this series. In a group of 31 pET patients treated by this conservative approach after a follow-up of at least 6 months, 10 patients were symptom-free after 6 weeks of training; 16 patients felt a significant reduction concerning intensity as well as frequency of their complaints, and thus, no further treatment was demanded. Patients acknowledged their own contributions with respect to their therapy.

Pearls

- *The patulous Eustachian tube (pET) is the result of an impaired protection function.*
- *The pET is confirmed by medical history.*
- *A passive Eustachian tube without an active muscular coordination should be absolutely avoided.*
- *The tensor veli palatini muscle and the medial pterygoid muscle have a common phylogenetic task.*
- *Aim of physiotherapy is the dynamic stabilization of hypo- or hyperfunctional craniomandibular and cervical muscles.*

Fig. 3.14 (a–c) Dynamic stabilization of the mandible. (**a**) Passive mobilization of mandibular joints. (**b**) Laterotrusion against a resistance. (**c**) Active jaw depression against a resistance

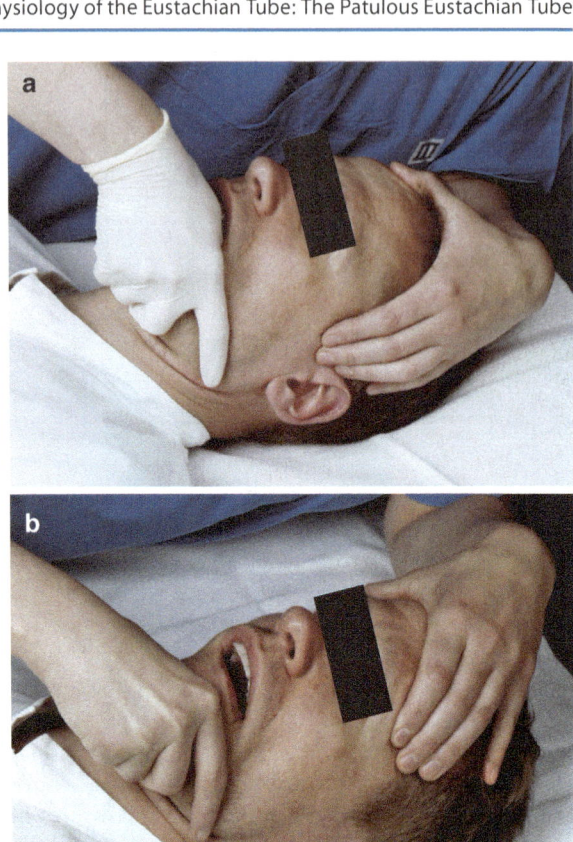

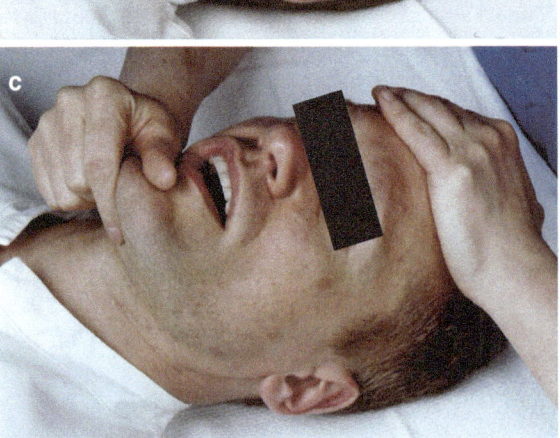

Fig. 3.15 Mobilization of the tongue against a resistance

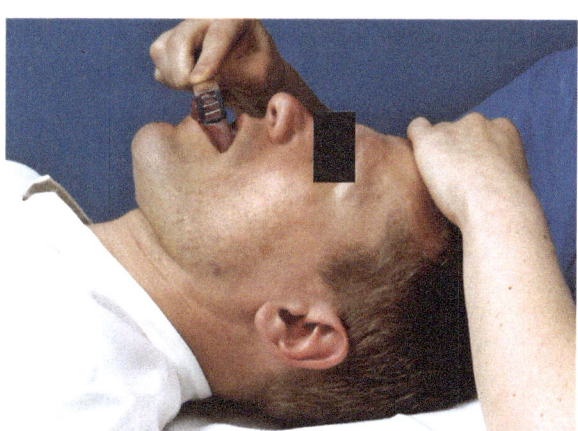

Tubal Function from a Middle Ear Surgeon's Viewpoint

4

- *Middle ear aeration: role of mucosa and ET*
- *Chronic middle ear disease*
- *Preoperative assessment*
- *Therapy of ET obstruction: balloon dilatation*
- *Principles of tympanoplasty*
- *Prognosis of surgery*

4.1 Eustachian Tube and Middle Ear Mucosa: Two Players that Are Not Well Understood

Good aeration of the middle ear space is a necessity for a well-functioning middle ear with regard to both infections and audiological function. Middle ear aeration is a result of a complex system involving at least two major contributors: the middle ear mucosa and the Eustachian tube [193]. Proper diagnoses of severe aeration problems and tube dysfunction are difficult because the system, its parts and their complex interaction are not fully understood.

Sadé and Ar [163] ascribe the major role of maintaining good aeration in the middle ear space to the middle ear mucosa. Examination of the middle ear reveals that those with good aeration have a well-aerated mastoid process whereas those with little aeration are characterized by contracted or poorly developed mastoids. The theory of the mucosa's contribution is supported by studies of total blockage of the Eustachian tube, which showed that continuous gas exchange in the middle ear space [192] is responsible for the continuous support of middle ear pressure. However, because the mucosa is too slow in following atmospheric pressure changes, this falls to the role of the Eustachian tube. In cases of acute and dramatic pressure changes, such as those that occur in diving or during an airplane flight, the Eustachian tube plays the additional role of an emergency valve. The Eustachian tube opens during procedures like swallowing, masticating and yawning, which help to in- or desufflate the middle ear space according to actual needs.

J.L. Dornhoffer et al., *A Practical Guide to the Eustachian Tube*,
DOI 10.1007/978-3-540-78638-2_4, © Springer-Verlag Berlin Heidelberg 2014

Classical tympanoplasty techniques solve mechanical problems, such as disrupted and fixed ossicular chains and perforated eardrums, but have little effect upon tubal dysfunction. There has been a trend towards surgical procedures that preserve the mucosa of the mastoid and antrum, with the concept that disruption of the mucosa is as counterproductive in temporal bone surgery as it is in sinus surgery. Thus, the surgical principle when treating chronic middle ear diseases is to support mucosal healing while restoring a closed middle ear space. In contrast to other surgical fields, it is not always possible to work in a noninfected environment in chronic otitis media as the surgery itself is conducted to achieve a dry, noninfected ear [212].

When dealing with the complex functional situation of the Eustachian tube and the middle ear mucosa, surgical solutions must deviate from pure mechanical manipulations, such as tympanoplasty. However, convincing results of the direct procedures suggested for Eustachian tube dysfunction are lacking. It is no wonder, then, that regardless of the large number of patients who experience Eustachian tube dysfunction and middle ear mucosa disorders, the number of patients in studies of direct Eustachian tube treatment is amazingly low.

4.1.1   General Assessment Prior to Middle Ear Surgery

Preoperative assessment includes a complete ENT examination. Of major interest is the situation in the nasopharynx, the soft palate, the lymphatic tissue, the adenoids and the tubal orifice and its surroundings. The extent of required imaging depends on the need for visualization of the disturbance. Although a plain radiograph (Schüller's view) can be obtained to get information on the middle ear space aeration status, CT scanning of the temporal bone affords more precise visualization. If information about the Eustachian tube's soft tissue is needed, MRI scanning is necessary. A complete audiometric evaluation, including pure tone and speech audiometry and speech discrimination, should be performed on all patients prior to middle ear surgery. The tuning fork examination according to Weber and Rinne is also necessary to confirm findings obtained in the audiogram.

4.1.2   Eustachian Tube: Preoperative Testing and Evaluation

Preoperative testing of Eustachian tube function is limited. The major clinical test for the Eustachian tube is Valsalva's manoeuvre [115,200,201]. The preoperative assessment before any ear surgery should include this simple tubal function test. If the patient is not able to perform the test, the variation according to Toynbee with a simultaneous swallowing manoeuvre may be helpful. Politzer's manoeuvre using the rubber balloon on the nostril when performing a k-plosive by the patient is more forceful but can still provide information about Eustachian tube patency. If the ear is Valsalva positive, then there is at least no mechanical blockage of the tube.

The patency of the Eustachian tube is most important regarding drainage function. Even if the situation for ventilation of the middle ear space is unclear, the Eustachian tube may still drain properly. A patient who is able to perform Valsalva's manoeuvre may be able to open his/her Eustachian tube postoperatively, and secretions from the middle ear can then be transported out of the middle ear space. However, this only indicates that there is an open passage; it is not a robust test of Eustachian tube function. Direct inflation using a tubal catheter [193], in our opinion, has no advantage, does not provide further information and is obviously more invasive.

4.2   Conservative Treatment of the Eustachian Tube Obstruction

Stangerup et al. [186] examined 45 children and 49 adults at Copenhagen Airport on 2 days in May 1995 for baro-otitis after landing. Barotrauma was classified otoscopically; middle ear pressure was assessed by tympanometry. About 25 % of the younger children suffered from baro-otitis. Whereas 21 % of these children were able to equilibrate their middle ear pressure by Valsalva's manoeuvre, 82 % could successfully increase middle ear pressure when using the Otovent™ treatment system for autoinflation.

4.3   Eustachian Tube Surgery: Tuboplasty Procedures – Bypass Surgery

A tuboplasty is any treatment directly impacting the Eustachian tube. Historically, there have been many tuboplasty procedures, including radioactive seed implantation (Sr-90), irradiation [164], bypass surgery (frontal sinus–middle ear, maxillary sinus–middle ear) [54] and tubal treatment via the middle fossa approach [71]. The tympano-oral conduit approach was performed in cadavers [88], and surgery creating a bypass parallel to the Eustachian tube was performed experimentally in dogs, followed by application in humans [121].

Many of these studies did not exceed the status of preliminary reports, and no major series were published. Other treatments, such as the Fulda aeration surgery [76] and similar procedures, demonstrate the multiple attempts to help patients with severe aeration problems. However, none of these extensive techniques has been proven in a major series.

4.3.1   Tubal Insertion

There have been several attempts to keep the lumen of the Eustachian tube open. Plastic catheters have been inserted, but the reports are only anecdotal and improvement lasted for only a short period of time [142]. Several publications from various

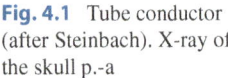

Fig. 4.1 Tube conductor (after Steinbach). X-ray of the skull p.-a

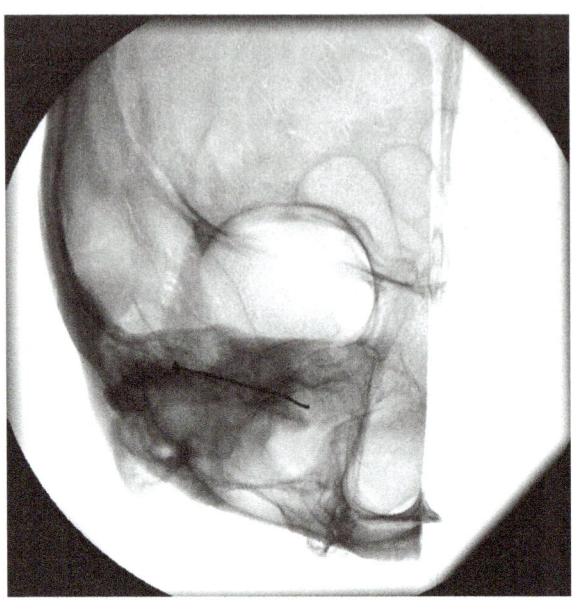

institutions describe the gold wire tube conductor introduced by Steinbach (Fig. 4.1). Lieberum and Jahnke [95] reported an increase of aeration after insertion of the wire in 11 out of 13 patients. Schrom et al. [171] inserted the gold wire in 125 patients, but 92 % showed no difference in tubal function after the procedure.

4.3.1.1   Balloon Dilatation of the Cartilaginous Portion

For cases of chronic obstructive Eustachian tube dysfunction, "balloon Eustachian tuboplasty" (BET) has been recently introduced by two different groups: the Bielefeld group [129] and the Boston group [144]. The method of dilatation of the cartilaginous part of the Eustachian tube has been proven feasible and safe in cadaver studies [112] and human adults [144]. Poe et al. [144] with their later study used their own catheter. In BET a balloon catheter is placed into the cartilaginous portion of the Eustachian tube by transnasal endoscopy-controlled insertion. The length of this balloon (*Bielefeld balloon catheter*, distribution by Spiggle and Theis®, Overath, Germany) with the Sudhoff group is 2 cm. This balloon is dilated up to 10 bar over a period of 2 min. With the dilation procedure, microfractures of the tubal cartilage with a successive expansion of the Rüdinger's safety canal could be experimentally observed, but the in vivo mechanism of the therapy remains unclear. Sudhoff and colleagues [190] treated 351 patients, of which the short-term results of 167 patients 2 months after the treatment and the long-term results of 53 patients 1 year after the treatment were recently published. They very thoroughly examined the pre- and postoperative Eustachian tube function using a modified manometry after the method of Estève. Depending on the relief with some of their patients, the dilation manoeuvre was repeated. According to their results, this procedure was satisfactory for 87 % of their patients. The Eustachian tube function tests were significantly better in more than 90 % of the cases.

4.3.2 Tubal Augmentation

The reports on augmentation surgery in the osseous part of the Eustachian tube are few. Steel probes were used to open soft tissue and osseous stenosis followed by palisade cartilage tympanoplasty, and good results were reported [63]. Charachon et al. [20] reported on a series of 17 patients in whom the osseous tube was opened and a silastic guide was inserted to keep the lumen patent. This could be achieved in nine ears. Extended tubotympanoplasty and drilling of the osseous part of the tube led to improvement in two of five patients in a study of Kumazawa et al. [87].

4.3.3 Laser Tuboplasty

Laser procedures have become popular in all fields of medicine. Laser treatment of the Eustachian tube is favoured as well. Success rates of laser tuboplasty are reported in up to 70 % of patients [86]. However, it should be noted that the laser treatment is directed towards the pharyngeal orifice or, additionally, the middle ear orifice of the Eustachian tube. It is no general treatment of the tube and does not encompass the mucosa/Eustachian tube system. Another issue with laser treatment is scarring. All procedures involving laser treatment lead to scarring to some extent; however, with regard to tubal function, this is a feared outcome as scarring is a major reason for dysfunction and tubal blocking.

4.3.4 The Unaerated Middle Ear: Total Stenosis of the Eustachian Tube

In cases of very reduced or no aeration of the middle ear space, Wullstein suggested type IV tympanoplasty. The main principle is to protect the round window from sound impact, so the sound wave enters the cochlea at the oval window solely. Absence of the tympanic membrane and ossicular chain leads to a conductive hearing loss of around 30 dB. Gerhardt [50] inserted an air-filled silicone bubble in the round window niche for better protection in type IV tympanoplasties. The type IV tympanoplasty may still be helpful in an atelectatic ear with or without cholesteatoma, providing a safe situation regarding infection but still bearing a large conductive hearing loss. Today, alternatives to the non-reconstructed middle ear mechanism exist in the form of bone-anchored or implantable hearing aids.

4.4 Eustachian Tube and Tympanoplasty

Tympanoplasty itself does not improve Eustachian tube function [68]. One main principle in tympanoplasty should always be to rely on the natural anatomical construction plan of the middle ear, so minimal changes should be made to help nature restore the middle ear's function [209]. If it is possible to leave the chain intact, ossicles should not be removed. A type I or type II tympanoplasty is preferred over techniques that require more extensive restorations, such as the type III tympanoplasty. Middle ear pressure should stabilize after 4 years, except in cases of cholesteatoma [202]. Alternatives to classical middle ear surgery using electrical hearing devices will be discussed at the end of this chapter.

4.4.1 Basic Considerations in Tympanoplasty. Two Main Goals: Eradication of Disease and Restoration of Hearing

The first aim of treatment in chronic middle ear disease is to cure the chronic inflammation. The risk of complications will depend on the entity of the middle ear disease. The most dangerous disease regarding infectious complications is undoubtedly cholesteatoma. Otogenic facial paresis, labyrinthitis, intracranial complications, sinus thrombosis, meningitis and epidural, subdural and brain abscess, when they occur, are regularly associated with cholesteatoma. The simple perforation of a mesotympanic otitis media may be recognized as less dangerous. A runny ear with slowly increasing hearing loss may be seen as a less dramatic situation, and the risk of life-threatening complications is negligible. Nevertheless, in the case of chronic suppurative otitis media or even with unspectacular chronic otitis media with effusion, all these major complications are possible.

The second aim in treating chronic middle ear disease is restoration of hearing. Since the beginning of modern tympanoplasty techniques in the 1950s, according to Moritz, Zöllner and Wullstein, attention has been recently more focused on hearing restoration techniques.

4.4.2 Materials for Reconstruction of the Tympanic Membrane

Many materials have been suggested for tympanic membrane reconstruction. Three tissues of autogenous origin are used today: temporal fascia (likely the material most favoured by surgeons all over the globe), perichondrium and cartilage [65]. Temporal fascia is easy to harvest and elegant to handle. Similar to fascia is perichondrium, which can be harvested either from the tragus or from the concha. Fascia and perichondrium are of similar resistance although some clinicians see advantages when using perichondrium [66]. Fascia and perichondrium are the materials of choice when the tympanic membrane is still cone-shaped because of the flexibility of the material. Fascia and perichondrium should be used in cases of primary surgery. In revision surgery cases and in atelectasis, a more resistant material is needed. Thus, cartilage is the material of choice for retraction pockets and atelectatic ears.

4.4.2.1 Harvesting Perichondrium and Cartilage

Cartilage and perichondrium are harvested either from the tragus or from the concha. The ideal region in the concha is the region of the cymba (Fig. 4.2a, b). In this area the cartilage is about 1 mm thick, and it is relatively flat with no disturbing connective tissue adhesions. An incision is made through the cartilage using a number 10 blade, and Metzenbaum scissors are used to remove the perichondrium,

Fig. 4.2 (**a**) Harvesting
cartilage from the concha
(cymba), cut through the
cartilage. (**b**) Preparation of
cymbal cartilage

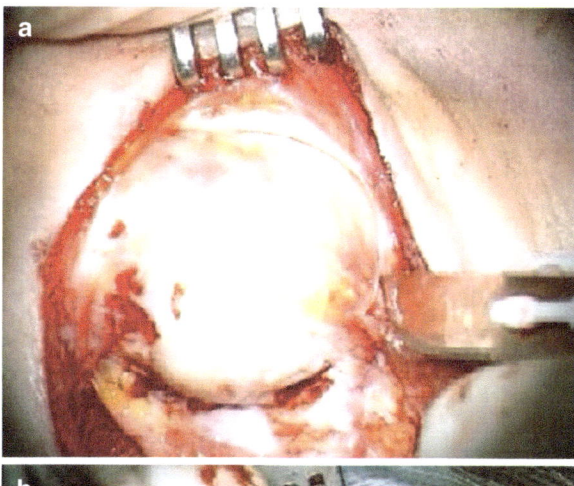

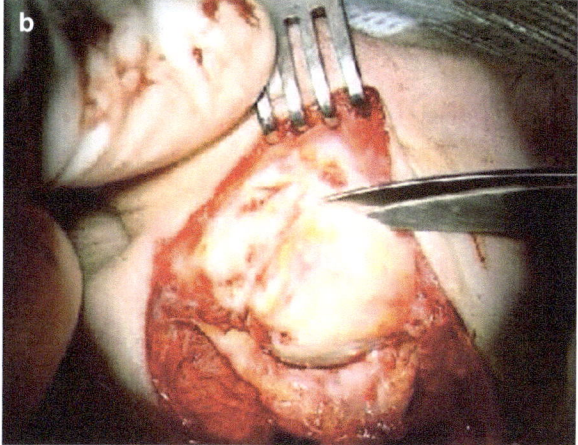

alone or attached to a piece of cartilage, leaving the anterior perichondrium in place. In a similar way, both materials can be harvested from the tragus. For cosmesis, the cut through the skin and cartilage should be performed about 2–3 mm beneath the free margin of the tragus (Fig. 4.3a, b). The cartilage can be used as a composite graft (cartilage/perichondrium island flap), as a cartilage plate or as shingles or palisades in a palisade technique [33,116].

4.4.2.2   Creating a Cartilage/Perichondrium Island Flap

To create a cartilage/perichondrium island flap, the cartilaginous margin of the harvested composite piece of cartilage and perichondrium is thinned using a number 10 blade. If using concha cartilage, the thinning is performed on the concave side, thus forcing the perichondrium fibres to bend the cartilage towards the opposite side and straightening the flap. The tragal cartilage may be slightly thinner and may not require this marginal trimming. The cartilage of the margin may then be removed with a Plester knife, thus creating a rim of perichondrium around the graft (Fig. 4.4). The acoustic properties of cartilage have been studied extensively by Zahnert and

Fig. 4.3 (**a**) Harvesting cartilage from the tragus. Cut should be 2 mm lower to the free margin for reasons of cosmesis. (**b**) Preparing tragal cartilage

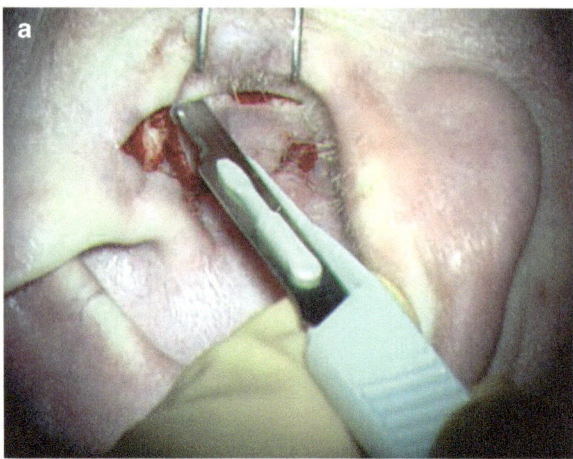

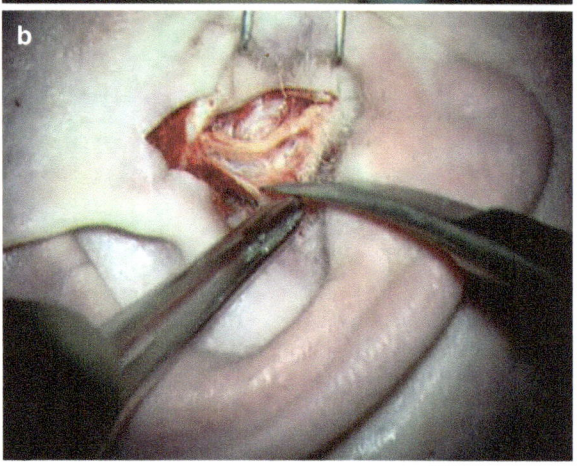

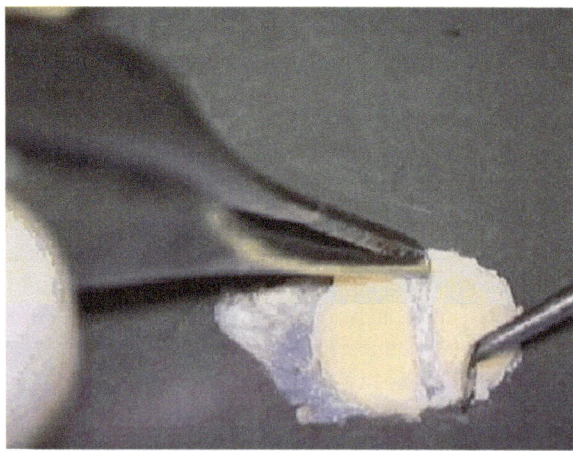

Fig. 4.4 Creating cartilage/perichondrium island. Notice rim in the middle for the malleus handle

Fig. 4.5 Cutting shingles

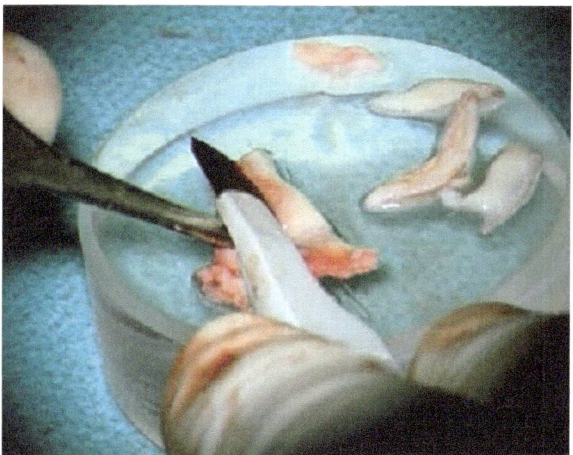

Fig. 4.6 Reconstruction of right tympanic membrane with palisades

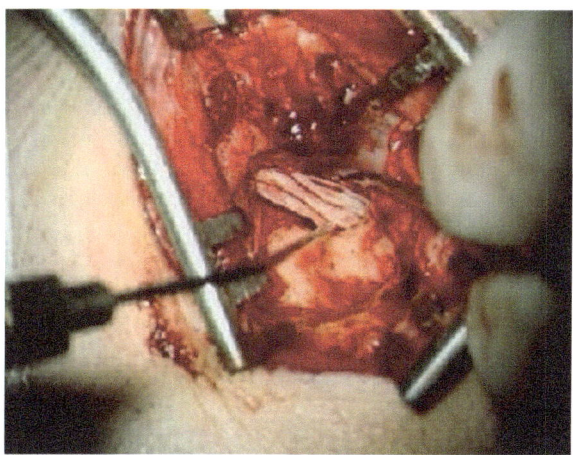

co-workers [215]. The results show that there is no obvious acoustical disadvantage using cartilage versus perichondrium or fascia, but the advantages in stability are enormous.

4.4.2.3   Palisade Technique

Heermann has used cartilage palisades since the late 1950s. The technique consists of placing longitudinal strips of cartilage parallel to the malleus handle while avoiding blockage of the orifice of the Eustachian tube in the middle ear [64]. The tympanic membrane reconstruction starts anteriorly, just above the opening of the Eustachian tube in the middle ear. Gaps between the palisades have to be avoided. It is helpful to cut the palisades like shingles and to pose them like shingles on a roof (Figs. 4.5 and 4.6).

Silastic sheeting of tympanic membrane and posterior wall reconstruction helps to avoid major granulation tissue growth in the early postoperative period (Fig. 4.7).

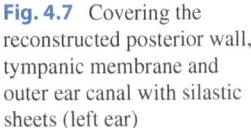
Fig. 4.7 Covering the reconstructed posterior wall, tympanic membrane and outer ear canal with silastic sheets (left ear)

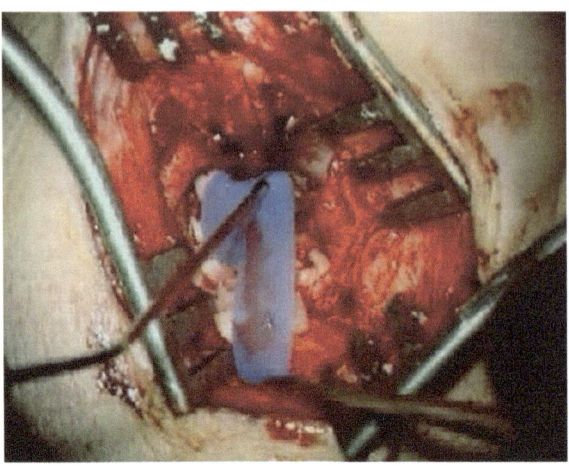

4.4.3   Materials for Reconstruction of the Ossicular Chain

A broad variety of materials are used for reconstruction of the ossicular chain. A patient's own material remains the gold standard. Autogenous ossicles, with the incus being the first choice, followed by the head of the malleus, are used with great acceptance. Adverse reactions from the implantation site are not expected. If the reconstruction is dislocated, there may be a problem with growth towards the promontory or the Fallopian canal, resulting in osseous fixation. Use of ossicles from ears with chronic otitis, where quite an amount of osteitis has been described histologically [46], is questionable. However, it is doubtful that the histological finding of osteitis is a problem for mechanical instability; rather, it may be the expression of the chronic otitis media itself. In cases of cholesteatoma, the use of a patient's own ossicles should be avoided in order to prevent recurrences.

Homogeneous ossicles have been widely used with satisfactory results regarding audiology and middle ear acceptance. However, because of the risk of transmitting viruses (HIV, hepatitis) and prions (Creutzfeldt–Jakob disease), the use of homogeneous ossicles has been almost completely abandoned. Heterogeneous materials are not used in middle ear surgery.

4.4.3.1   Alloplastic Materials

Since the origination of tympanoplasty, alloplastic materials have been used extensively and uncritically. However, as the biology of the implantation site in the middle ear has become better understood, both biocompatible and unacceptable materials have emerged. These are listed in Table 4.1. The majority of acceptable materials are fashioned from hydroxyapatite, high-density porous ethylene and titanium (Fig. 4.8a, b).

Despite histological studies showing adverse reaction to ethylene, high-density porous ethylene seems to be acceptable as ossicle prosthesis material. The majority

Table 4.1 Materials for middle ear prostheses (selection)	Stapes surgery	Platinum–Teflon® (polytetrafluorethylene)
		Titanium
		Stainless steel
		Gold
	Chronic middle ear disease	Titanium
		Aluminium oxide
		Bioverit®
		Glassionomeric cement
		Hydroxyapatite–polyethylene, hydroxyapatite
		Gold
		Stainless steel

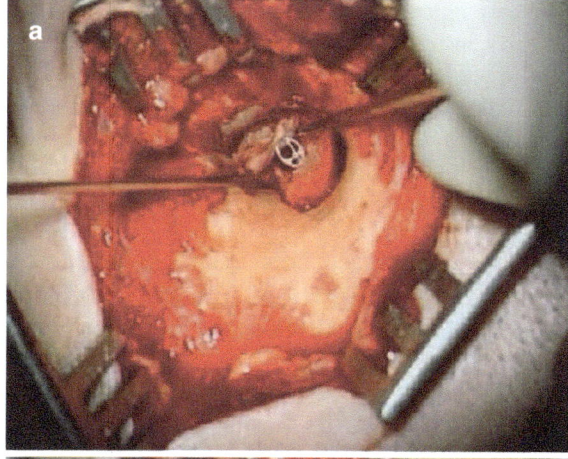

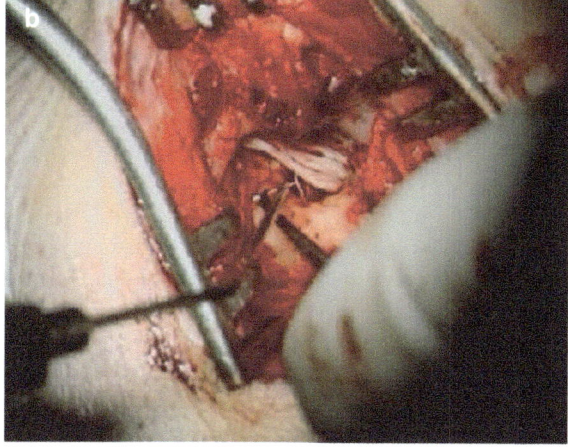

Fig. 4.8 (**a**) Positioning of prosthesis underneath tympanic membrane (left ear). (**b**) Reconstructed canal wall posterior to position of prosthesis underneath palisades, right (right ear)

of prostheses used today are constructed of hydroxyapatite, titanium or a composite of both. Each of these biocompatible materials has advantages and disadvantages. Hydroxyapatite can be moulded in the production process, reducing sharp edges that can lead to protrusion, but it is slightly heavier of the two materials and non-malleable. Within the last 10 years, titanium has gained more popularity in Europe due to its biocompatibility and its light weight. Its malleability allows formation into filigree-type prostheses that do not compromise the gas space in the middle ear. It does, however, have sharp edges, requiring the placement of a small piece of cartilage on top of the prosthesis to ensure stability against the reconstructed eardrum. Because of the common atelectasis phenomenon in the chronically diseased middle ear, there is always a tendency of protrusion of the prostheses. Therefore, when using the palisade technique, it is important to provide complete coverage of the prosthesis with the cartilage pieces.

4.4.3.2 Protrusion or Extrusion?

The terms protrusion and extrusion may be used interchangeably, but the surgeon should consider these to be different processes. In chronic middle ear disease, the tendency of atelectasis is common. That means protrusion of the ossicular chain is part of the natural course of the diseases. The term extrusion should be related to an active process and should be distinguishable histologically. Active cellular signs of rejection, like giant foreign body cells, should be found when using the term extrusion.

4.5 Eustachian Tube Function in Different Middle Ear Disease Entities and Consequences for Surgical Treatment

4.5.1 Chronic Otitis Media with Effusion

Chronic otitis media with effusion is the typical disease of young children, the major age group experiencing this condition being between 4 and 6 years. It typically results from the combination of recurrent middle ear effusion, adenoid hypertrophy and, often, hyperplasia of the tonsils. The underlying condition is obstruction of the nasal passages, so typically these children breathe through their mouths. The adenoids not only block the nasal airway, but they also are the reason for recurrent infections as they host a reservoir of bacteria. Paracentesis and suction of the effusion, followed by placement of tympanostomy tubes, is a widespread treatment. However, tympanostomy tubes, since they are foreign bodies, may lead to tissue non-acceptance and even adverse reactions, such as permanent otorrhea. Therefore, this should not be the treatment of choice in a primary situation.

In adenoid hyperplasia with obstruction of the nose, a situation that hinders not only the aeration of the ear but also the aeration of the sinuses, the mechanical blockage should be removed. Gates et al. [49] showed significant advantage of adenoidectomy combined with paracentesis versus tympanostomy tubes alone or in combination with adenoidectomy. Most of the children with these conditions then need no further treatment. In the case of major tonsillar hyperplasia (e.g. "kissing" tonsils), tonsillectomy may also be indicated. If there is no history of tonsillitis, laser tonsillotomy can be considered. Accompanying Eustachian tube inflating procedures are helpful. If Valsalva's manoeuvre cannot be performed by younger patients, an alternative is the Otovent® balloon manoeuvre. By inflating an air balloon via one nostril while the opposite one is compressed, an insufflation of the middle ear is possible. If all these surgical and non-surgical therapies fail, the recommendation is to insert tympanometry tubes. Directly treating the Eustachian tube is not helpful and should be avoided, especially in children.

4.5.2   Chronic Suppurative Otitis Media

The situation in chronic suppurative otitis media is characterized by a central perforation. There are periods of a runny ear followed by times of no discharge. X-ray imaging of the temporal bone may show reduced aeration of the mastoid. It is not unusual for Valsalva's manoeuvre to be negative. In those situations, the risk of reperforation is high. The perforation itself seems to function as a natural tympanostomy tube. Fascia or perichondrium can be used in primary surgery; in revision cases, cartilage is recommended.

4.5.3   Atelectatic Ear (Adhesive Process)

The aetiology of the atelectatic ear is still unclear. The finding may be a retraction in the posterior part of the tympanic membrane deep into both niches and the hypotympanum, with the anterior part of the tympanic membrane appearing normal. The Eustachian tube may be inflatable (Valsalva positive), or the manoeuvre may be negative. It is unclear why only parts of the eardrum retract. In an open, communicating, gas-filled space, the pressure should be the same everywhere. There may be mucosa folds that separate different compartments, or the resistance of the tympanic membrane may be different due to recurrent infections and perforations.

In treating this condition, ventilation procedures should be considered (e.g. Valsalva's manoeuvre, Otovent® balloon insufflation in children) (Fig. 4.9). If these conservative procedures fail, surgery is recommended. The surgical treatment consists of removing all the retracted epithelium of the tympanic membrane. This type of surgery is one of the most delicate operations in the middle ear. If keratinized squamous epithelium is left, an iatrogenic cholesteatoma will result. The Eustachian tube may be probed, and at least the middle ear orifice should be inspected. Tube probing should be done very gently and should not be forced at any time. The reconstruction of the tympanic membrane in these ears needs resistant material, and cartilage is the material of choice. Tympanosclerotic plaques should be removed, but mucosa should be saved as much as possible. If the tympanic membrane does not perforate and the aeration of the tympanum remains stable, there is a chance of

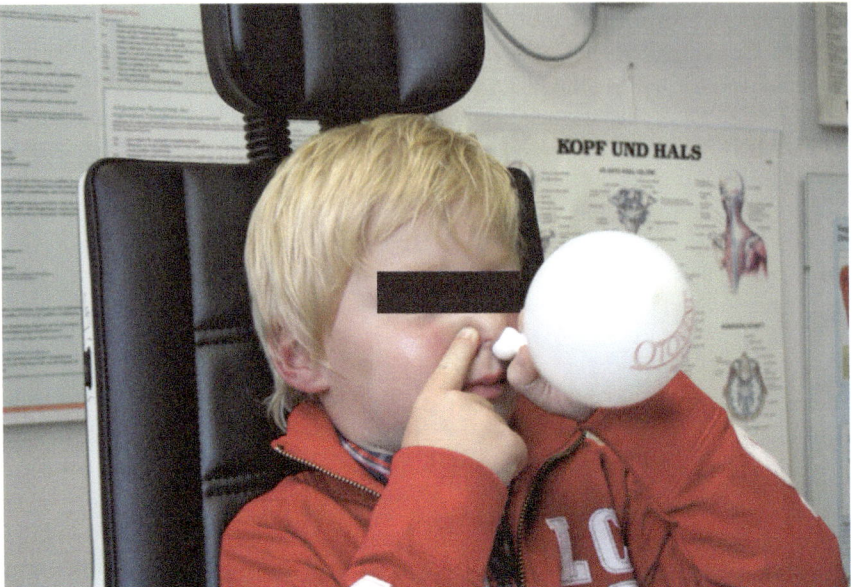

Fig. 4.9 Valsalva's manoeuvre assisted by using the Otovent® balloon

healing. Besides stapes surgery, which has to be postponed to ensure the creation of an aerated, non-inflamed process, ossicular chain reconstruction should be performed during the primary operation.

4.5.4 Tympanosclerosis and Tympanofibrosis

If the perforation in chronic suppurative otitis media exists over a long time and periods of recurrent inflammation occur, there will be an increasing deposit of calcified tympanosclerotic plaques. Often this tympanosclerotic process leads to ankylosis of the ossicular chain. If necessary, the malleus and incus are removed with no major risk. Mobilization of the stapes should be avoided because of the risk of labyrinthine fistula, followed by labyrinthitis and deafness. If an attempt is planned to treat the fixation-related hearing loss, a stapedectomy is performed. This is less risky when the eardrum is closed and an abacterial environment has been restored.

4.5.5 Cholesteatoma

In cases of cholesteatoma, keratinizing squamous epithelium is in the middle ear space, where non-keratinizing squamous epithelium (mucosa) usually exists. The rare and totally different situation of displaced epithelium in congenital

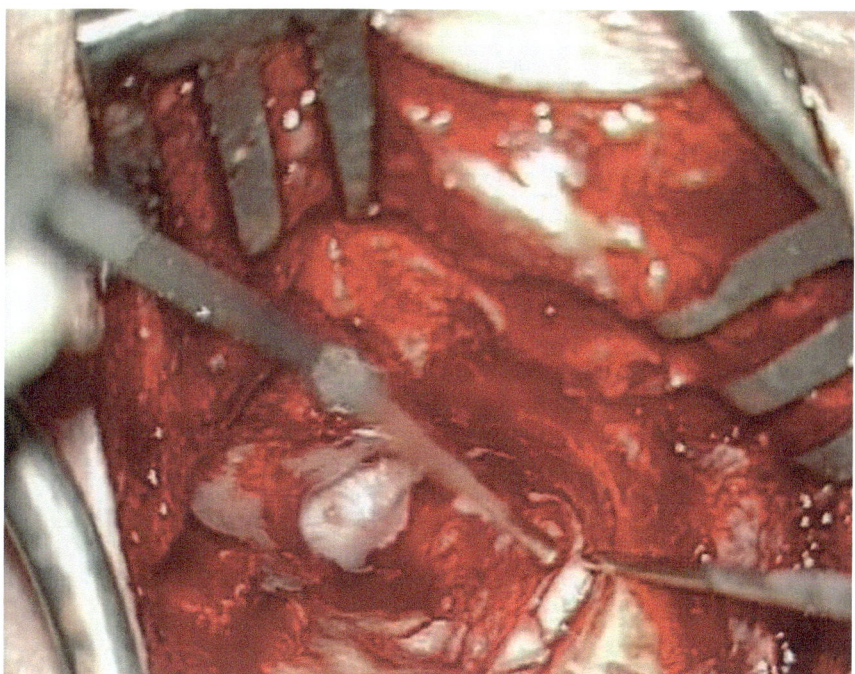

Fig. 4.10 Reconstruction of posterior wall with cartilage after cholesteatoma removal in a canal-wall-down procedure (left ear). Anterior tympanic membrane intact

cholesteatoma is beyond the scope of this discussion, as it is not related to tubal dysfunction. From the clinical standpoint, there are at least two entities of acquired cholesteatoma: the classical cholesteatoma of the pars flaccida (epitympanic cholesteatoma) and the pars tensa cholesteatoma (mesotympanic cholesteatoma).

Whether sniffing is a major contributor to cholesteatoma development is still a controversy. Incidences of 25–82 % have been reported [83,103]; others found sniffing to be the cause in at least 50 % of acquired cholesteatoma cases [193]. In our opinion, sniffing-induced cholesteatoma may be overestimated.

4.5.5.1   Epitympanic Cholesteatoma

The typical cholesteatoma is an epitympanal retraction pocket, growing onion-like towards the antrum and mastoid. The tympanum itself is aerated, and Valsalva's manoeuvre is often positive. Probing of the Eustachian tube in most patients is possible, and the mastoid may be well aerated. Techniques for cholesteatoma removal should have a low risk of recurrence or residual disease. The favoured technique is a canal-wall-down technique [66,67], in which the cholesteatoma can be traced from its origin in the middle ear and tracked into the antrum and mastoid. Following the basic rule of restoring the natural situation, the posterior wall is then reconstructed (Fig. 4.10). Many materials have been suggested for this, including bone plates, different types of cement and titanium [51,189]. Cartilage has major

Fig. 4.11 Second-look surgery of right ear, partial prosthesis at 4 o'clock. Cochleariform process and tensor tympani tendon (middle)

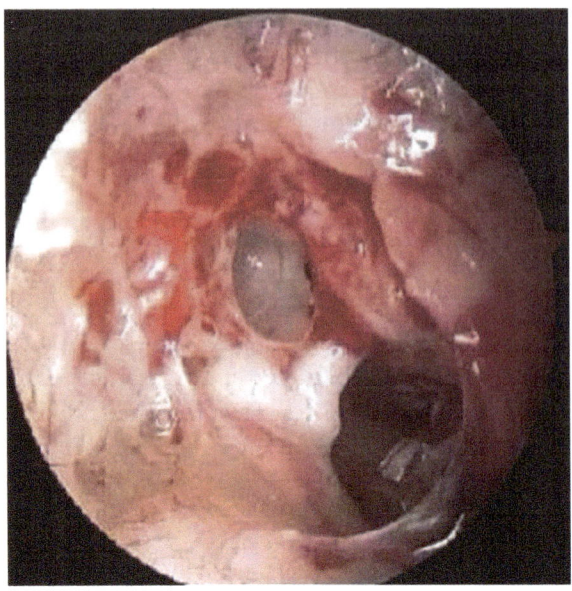

advantages as it is available in sufficient amounts, is stable and has excellent healing and biocompatibility properties. Cholesteatoma removal and reconstruction of the ossicular chain and tympanic membrane are performed as a single-stage procedure. Exceptions are subluxations of the stapes and footplate, fractures or perilymph fistulas. If the surgeon has any doubt that there may be some remnant of keratinizing epithelium, there will be a need for second-look surgery (Fig. 4.11).

4.5.5.2 Mesotympanic Cholesteatoma

Mesotympanic, or pars tensa, cholesteatoma results from atelectasis and is located in the posterior quadrants of the tympanic membrane and tympanum. These cholesteatomas grow very deep medially to the Fallopian canal and into the barely visible area of the sinus tympani. Meticulous removal of all keratinizing epithelium is necessary. To ensure that no epithelium remains, the tympanum mirror according to Heermann is used or Hopkins telescopes are helpful.

4.5.6 Eustachian Tube Function, Eradication of Sinonasal Disease, Adenoidectomy and Tympanoplasty

Influences of the nasal airway on Eustachian tube function and, thus, the middle ear may be assumed but have not been proven scientifically. Regardless, upper airway obstruction by adenoids, hyperplastic tonsils or major deviations of the nasal septum need to be corrected prior to middle ear surgery. The time period between the nasal or pharyngeal procedure and the middle ear treatment should be at least 3 months and, preferably, 6 months. Most patients suffering from chronic sinus disease have no Eustachian tube or middle ear problems. In cases of combined problems, however, eradication of sinus disease should be performed first, and the period of time prior to tympanoplasty should be at least 6 months.

4.6   Prediction of Tympanoplasty Results, Eustachian Tube Function and Aeration Status

A prediction of the prognosis of tympanoplasty based on Eustachian tube function tests is impossible. It is also impossible to determine normal Eustachian tube function based on the results of tympanoplasty. To date, there is no reliable test to determine the interaction of these factors on outcome [115]. In one study, mastoid cell aeration, Eustachian tube function and tympanoplasty results showed no interdependence, so prediction was not possible [179,180]. In cleft palate patients, poor Eustachian tube function is assumed. However, one study showed no statistical difference in the postoperative outcome comparing patients with repaired cleft palate to non-cleft patients [48].

4.6.1   Eustachian Tube Function and Mastoid Surgery

Mastoidectomy in combination with tympanoplasty is widely used, even in noncholesteatoma cases. However, mastoidectomy does not improve the aeration situation in the middle ear space. Takahashi [192] showed that a postmastoidectomy cavity could not be expected to revive as a functioning gas exchange chamber. Usually the cavity is filled with scar tissue after mastoidectomy. Even in situations such as re-saccotomy, where totally normal gas function in the middle ear can be expected, some amounts of scarring will be regularly found.

The benefit of tympanoplasty in combination with mastoidectomy is questionable. Balyan et al. [8], Mishiro et al. [119] and Albu et al. [2] found no statistical difference comparing two cohorts, one receiving tympanoplasty with mastoidectomy and one without mastoidectomy. McGrew at al. [114] reported an advantage with additional mastoid surgery, but this was not statistically proven.

4.6.2   Ventilation Tubes, Tympanoplasty and Eustachian Tube Dysfunction

In some situations, because of the inability to measure Eustachian tube function preoperatively, the postoperative course after reconstruction of the tympanic membrane may be complicated by effusion, leading to less than satisfactory hearing results. Every attempt should be made to improve tubal function, via Valsalva's manoeuvre or Otovent® balloon insufflation in children, and to eradicate sinunasal disease. However, a certain percentage of patients will continue, in spite of these efforts, to experience effusion and conductive hearing loss. In these cases, one must weigh the benefits and risks of tympanostomy tubes, which will improve hearing but may lead to recurrent drainage. Furthermore, it has been suggested that ventilating the reconstructed tympanic membrane will facilitate healing of the middle ear mucosa after tympanoplasty [200].

4.7 Alternatives for the Unaerated Middle Ear: Conventional Hearing Aid, Bone-Anchored Hearing Aid (BAHA) and Implantable Hearing Aid

Resulting hearing deficits after tympanoplasty may require the use of hearing aids. Classical air-conducting aids may be suggested. However, if the ear has recurrent drainage due to a canal-wall-down surgery, plugging the canal with hearing aids will impair the situation. Bone-conducting hearing aids are then indicated. The bone-anchored hearing aid (BAHA) was developed for patients with conductive hearing loss and normal or near-normal inner ear function. This is a typical situation of ears with bad aeration missing Eustachian tube and mucosal gas exchange function. In cases of major conductive hearing loss, new indications for implantable hearing aids, developed for patients with sensorineural hearing loss, have been implemented [80]. Following an idea published by Spindel et al. [185], Colletti [23] clinically introduced a new indication for the semi-implantable Vibrant Soundbridge® device, suggesting placement of the floating mass transducer directly at the round window. Depending on the extent of sensorineural hearing deficit the Vibrant Bonebridge® avoids further manipulations in the middle ear cavity. In cases where classical tympanoplasty techniques result in a hearing deficit, these alternatives should all be considered.

Pearls

- *Continuous gas exchange in the middle ear space contributes to the static the middle ear pressure.*
- The *principle of middle ear surgery is to support mucosal healing.*
- *The Bielefeld balloon catheter is a promising tool for the treatment of chronic obstructive ET dysfunction, but its* in vivo *effect remains unclear.*
- *Follow-the-pathology is the favoured technique for cholesteatoma surgery.*
- *Mastoidectomy does not improve the aeration of the middle ear space.*

References

1. Akita K, Shimokawa T, Sato T (2003) An anatomic study of the positional relationships between the lateral pterygoid muscle and its surrounding nerves. Eur J Anat 7(suppl 1):5–14
2. Albu S, Trabalzini F, Amadori M (2012) Usefulness of cortical mastoidectomy in myringoplasty. Otol Neurotol 33:604–609
3. Allen GW (1967) Abnormal patency of the Eustachian tube. A complication of oral contraception. JAMA 200:412–413
4. Amoodi H, Bance M, Thamboo A (2010) Magnetic resonance imaging illustrating change in the ostmann fat pad with age. J Otolaryngol Head Neck Surg 39:440–441
5. Aschan G (1955) The anatomy of the Eustachian tube with regard to its function. Acta Soc Med Ups 60:131–149
6. Asenov DR, Nath V, Telle A, Antweiler C, Walther LE, Vary P, Di Martino E (2010) Sonotubometry with perfect sequences: first results in pathological ears. Acta Otolaryngol 130:1242–1248
7. Baarsma EA (2006) Bartolomeo Eustachi. Ned Tijdschr KNO-Heelk 12:95–99
8. Balyan FR, Celikkanat S, Aslan A et al (1997) Mastoidectomy in noncholesteatomatous chronic suppurative otitis media: is it necessary? Otolaryngol Head Neck Surg 117:592–595
9. Barsoumian R, Kuehn DP, Moon JB, Canady JW (1998) An anatomic study of the tensor veli palatini and dilator tubae muscles in relation to Eustachian tube and velar function. Cleft Palate Craniofac J 35:101–110
10. Bartlett C, Pennings R, Ho A, Kirkpatrick D, Wijhe R, Bance M (2010) Simple mass loading of the tympanic membrane to alleviate symptoms of patulous Eustachian tube. J Otolaryngol Head Neck Surg 39:259–268
11. Bluestone CD (1983) Eustachian tube function: physiology, pathophysiology, and role of allergy in pathogenesis of otitis media. J Allergy Clin Immunol 72:242–251
12. Bluestone CD (2005) Eustachian tube: structure, function, role in otitis media. BC Decker, Hamilton
13. Bluestone CD, Cantekin EI (1981) Management of the patulous Eustachian tube. Laryngoscope 91:149–152
14. Buetow KW, Louw B, Hugo SR, Grimbeeck RJ (1991) Tensor veli palatini muscle tension sling for eustachian tube function in cleft palate. Surgical technique and audiometric examination. J Craniomaxillofac Surg 19(2):71–76
15. Bunne M, Magnuson B, Falk B, Hellström S (2000) Eustachian tube function varies over time in children with secretory otitis media. Acta Otolaryngol 120:716–723
16. Bryant WS (1907) The Eustachian tube, its anatomy and its movement: with a description of the cartilages, muscles, fasciae, and the fossa of Rosenmüller. Med Rec 71:931–934
17. Bylander A (1980) Comparison of eustachian tube function in children and adults with normal ear. Ann Otol Rhinol Laryngol 89(suppl 68):20–24
18. Cantekin E, Doyle WJ, Reichert TJ, Phillips DC, Bluestone CD (1979) Dilation of the Eustachian tube by electrical stimulation of the mandibular nerve. Ann Otol 88:40–51

19. Ceylan A, Göksu N, Kemaloglu YK, Ugur B, Akyürek N, Bayazik YA (2007) Impact of Jacobson's (tympanic) nerve sectioning on middle ear functions. Otol Neurotol 28:341–344

20. Charachon R, Gratacap B, Lerat M (1986) Chirurgie de la trompe d'Eustache osseuse et de l'isthme tubaire. Rev Laryngol 107:45–48

21. Chen DA, Luxford WM (1990) Myringotomy and tube for relief of patulous eustachian tube symptoms. Am J Otol 11:272–273

22. Cheng PW, Young YH, Lou PJ (1999) Patulous Eustachian tube in long-term survivors of nasopharyngeal carcinoma. Ann Otol Rhinol Laryngol 108(2):201–204

23. Colletti V, Soli SD, Carner M, Colletti L (2006) Treatment of mixed hearing losses via implantation of a vibratory transducer on the round window. Int J Audiol 45:600–608

24. Corbeel L (2007) What is new in otitis media. Eur J Pediatr 166:511–519

25. Cox JR (1980) Hormonal influence on auditory function. Ear Hearing 1:219–222

26. Dayan JH, Smith D, Oliker A, Haring J, Cutting CB (2005) A virtual reality model of Eustachian tube dilation and clinical implications for cleft palate repair. Plast Reconstr Surg 116:236–241

27. De la Cuadra Blanco C, Peces Peña MD, Rodríguez-Vázquez JF, Mérida-Velasco JA, Mérida-Velasco JR (2012) Development of the human tensor veli palatini: specimens measuring 13.6–137 mm greatest length; weeks 6–16 of development. Cells Tissues Organs 195:392–399

28. DiBartolomeo JR, Henry DF (1992) A new medication to control patulous Eustachian tube disorders. Am J Otol 13:323–327

29. DiMartino E, Thaden R, Krombach GA, Westhofen M (2004) Funktionsuntersuchungen der Tuba Eustachii. Aktueller Stand HNO 52:1029–1040

30. DiMartino E, Walther LE, Westhofen M (2005) Endoscopic examination of the Eustachian tube: a step-by-step approach. Otol Neurotol 26:1112–1117

31. Doherty JK, Slattery WH (2003) Autologous fat grafting for the refractory patulous Eustachian tube. Otolaryngol Head Neck Surg 128:88–91

32. Domenech-Ratto G (1977) Development and peripheral innervation of the palatal muscles. Acta Anat Basel 97(1):4–14

33. Dornhoffer J (2003) Cartilage tympanoplasty: indications, techniques, and outcomes in a 1,000-patient series. Laryngoscope 113(11):1844–1856

34. Doyle WJ (2002) The link between allergic rhinitis and otitis media. Curr Opin Allergy Clin Immunol 2:21–25

35. Doyle WJ, Rood SR (1980) Comparison of the anatomy of the Eustachian tube in the rhesus monkey (Macaca mulatta) and man: implications for physiologic modeling. Ann Otol Rhinol Laryngol 89:49–57

36. Doyle WJ, Swarts JD (2010) Eustachian tube–Tensor veli palatini muscle–cranial base relationships in children and adults: an osteological study. Int J Pediatr Otorhinolaryngol 74:986–990

37. Dyer RK, McElveen JT (1991) The patulous Eustachian tube: management options. Otolaryngol Head Neck Surg 105:832–835

38. Eden AR, Gannon PJ (1987) Neural control of middle ear aeration. Arch Otolaryngol Head Neck Surg 113:133–137

39. Estève D, Dubreuil C, Della Vedova C, Normand B, Martin C (2001) Evaluation par tubo-manometrie de la function d'ouverture tubaire et de la réponse tympanique chez le sujet normal et chez le sujet porteur d'une otide séro-muqueuse chronique: comparaison des resultats. J Fr ORL 50:223–231

40. Feldmann H (1996) The Eustachian tube and its part in the history of otology. Laryngo-Rhino-Otol 75:783–792

41. Finkelstein Y, Talmi YP, Rubel Y, Zohar Y (1988) An objective method for evaluation of the patulous Eustachian tube by using the middle ear analyzer. Arch Otolaryngol Head Neck Surg 114:1134–1138

42. Finkelstein Y, Talmi YP, Nachmani A, Hauben D, Zohar Y (1989) Pathology of levator veli palatini muscle and Eustachian tube. In: Conference of the Eustachian tube and middle ear diseases, Geneva

43. Finkelstein Y, Wexler DB, Nachmani A, Ophir D (2002) Endoscopic partial adenoidectomy for children with submucous cleft palate. Cleft Palate Craniofac J 39:479–486
44. Flisberg K, Ingelstedt S (1969) Middle-ear mechanics in patulous tube cases. Acta Otolaryngol (Stockh) (Suppl) 263:18–22
45. Flores RL, Jones BL, Bernstein J, Karnell M, Canady J, Cutting CB (2010) Tensor veli palatini preservation, transection, and transection with tensor tenopexy during cleft palate repair and its effects on Eustachian tube function. Plast Reconstr Surg 125:282–289
46. Frese KA, Hoppe F (1996) Morphologische Untersuchungen an autologen und homologen Ossikeln nach Langzeitimplantation. Laryngo-Rhino-Otol 75:330–334
47. Gannon PJ, Eden AR, Laitman JT (1994) Functional compartments of the tensor veli palatini muscle. Arch Otolaryngol Head Neck Surg 120:1382–1389
48. Gardner E, Dornhoffer J (2002) Tympanoplasty results in patients with cleft palate: an age- and procedure-matched comparison of preliminary results with patients without cleft palate. Otolaryngol Head Neck Surg 5:518–523
49. Gates GA, Avery CA, Prihoda TJ et al (1987) Effectiveness of adenoidectomy and tympanostomy tubes in the treatment of chronic otitis media with effusion. N Engl J Med 317:1444–1451
50. Gerhardt HJ (1972) Operative Hörverbesserung bei verödetem Mittelohr und irreversibel verschlossener Tube (1. Mitteilung). Acta Otolaryngol 74:57–60
51. Geyer G, Städtgen A, Schwager K, Jonck L (1998) Ionomeric cement implants in the middle ear of the baboon (Papio ursinus) as a primate model. Eur Arch Otorhinolaryngol 255(8):402–409
52. Ghadiali SN, Banks J, Swarts JD (2004) Finite element analysis of active Eustachian tube function. J Appl Physiol 97:648–654
53. Ghadiali SN, Swarts JD, Doyle WJ (2003) Effect of tensor veli palatini paralysis on Eustachian tube mechanics. Ann Otol Rhinol Laryngol 112:704–711
54. Goode R, Glasscock M (1974) The tympano-frontal shunt: a procedure for the treatment of chronic Eustachian Tube insufficiency. Laryngoscope 85:100–112
55. Grant HR, Quiney RE, Mercer DM, Lodge S (1988) Cleft palate and glue ear. Arch Dis Child 63:176–179
56. Guild SR (1956) Elastic tissue of the Eustachian tube. Ann Otol Rhinol Laryngol 64:537–543
57. Guindi GM, Charia KKC (1980) A reappraisal of the salpingo-pharyngeus muscle. Arch Otorhinolaryngol 229:135–141
58. Handzel O, Poe D, Marchbanks RJ (2012) Synchronous endoscopy and sonotubometry of the Eustachian tube: a pilot study. Otol Neurotol 33:184–191
59. Handzic-Cuk J, Cuk V, Gluhinic M, Risavi R, Stajner-Katusic S (2001) Tympanometric findings in cleft palate patients: influence of age and cleft type. J Laryngol Otol 115:91–96
60. Hauser R, Münker G (1989) Sniff-induzierter Unterdruck – eine Ursache für die Entstehung von Mittelohrerkrankungen? HNO 37:242–247
61. Hecht CS, Gannon PJ, Eden AR (1993) Motor innervation of the Eustachian tube muscles in the Guinea pig. Laryngoscope 103:1218–1226
62. Heermann J (1988) Einseitig weite Tuba auditiva mit Tinnitus, Innenohrschaden, Schwindel und Hörsturz – Collageninjektion. HNO 36:13–15
63. Heermann J, Heermann H, Heermann P (1973) Konisch-ovale Stahlsonden zur Weitung oder Fraktur knöcherner Stenosen der Tuba Eustachii. Z Laryngol Rhinol Otol Grenzgebiete 52:578–582
64. Heermann J Jr, Heermann H, Kopstein E (1970) Fascia and cartilage palisade tympanoplasty. Nine years' experience. Arch Otolaryngol 91:228–241
65. Helms J (1983) Die Wiederherstellung der Schalleitungskette. HNO 31:37–44
66. Helms J (1995) Moderne Aspekte der Tympanoplastik. Laryngo-Rhino-Otol 74:465–467
67. Hildmann H, Sudhoff H (2006) Middle ear surgery. Springer, Berlin/Heidelberg/New York
68. Holmquist J (1991) Eustachian tube function and tympanoplasty. Acta Otorhinolaryngol Belg 45:67–69

69. Honjo I (1988) Eustachian tube and middle ear diseases: middle ear disease and Eustachian tube in patients with cleft palate. Springer, Tokyo

70. Honjo I, Ushiro K, Okazaki N, Kumazawa T (1981) Evaluation of Eustachian tube function by contrast roentgenography. Arch Otolaryngol 107:350–352

71. House W, Glasscock M, Miles J (1969) Eustachian tuboplasty. Laryngoscope 79: 1765–1782

72. Hubbard BA, Rice GB, Muzaffar AR (2010) Adenoid involvement in velopharyngeal closure in children with cleft palate. Can J Plast Surg 18:135–138

73. Ishijima K, Sando I, Balaban CD, Miura M, Takasaki K (2002) Functional anatomy of the levator veli palatine muscle and tensor veli palatine muscle in association with Eustachian tube cartilage. Ann Otol Rhinol Laryngol 111:530–536

74. Iwano T, Kinoshita T, Hamada E, Ushiro K, Yamashita T, Kumazawa T (1991) Sensation of ear fullness caused by Eustachian tube dysfunction. Auris Nasus Larynx 18(4):343–349

75. Iwano T, Ushiro K, Yukawa N, Doi T, Kinoshita T, Hamada E, Kumazawa T (1993) Active opening function of the human Eustachian tube: comparison between sonotubometry and pressure equilibration test. Acta Otolaryngol (Stockh) (Suppl) 500:62–65

76. Kaftan H, Draf W (2000) "Fuldaer Belüftungsoperation" – ein operatives Konzept bei ausgeprägten Ventilationsstörungen des Mittelohres. Laryngo-Rhino-Otol 79:8–13

77. Kane AA, Lo LJ, Yen BD, Chen YR, Noordhoff MS (2000) The effect of hamulus fracture on the outcome of palatoplasty: a preliminary report of a prospective, alternating study. Cleft Palate Craniofac J 37:506–511

78. Kapur TR (1995) Causes of failure of combined approach tympanoplasty in the treatment of acquired cholesteatomas of the middle ear and the mastoid. J Laryngol Otol 109:710–712

79. Karwautz A, Hafferl A, Ungar D, Sailer H (1999) Patulous Eustachian tube in a case of adolescent anorexia nervosa. Int J Eat Disord 25(3):353–356

80. Kitahara M, Kodama A, Ozawa H, Izukura H, Inoue S (1994) Pressure test in normal subjects. Acta Otolaryngol (Stockh) (Suppl) 510:104–106

81. Kiefer J, Arnold W, Staudenmaier R (2006) Round window stimulation with an implantable hearing aid (Soundbridge®) combined with autogenous reconstruction of the auricle – a new approach. ORL 68:378–385

82. Klockars T, Rautio J (2012) Early placement of ventilation tubes in cleft lip and palate patients: does palatal closure affect tube occlusion and short-term outcome? Int J Pediatr Otorhinolaryngol 76:1481–1484

83. Kobayashi T, Yaginuma Y, Takahashi Y, Takasaka T (1996) Incidence of sniff-induced cholesteatoma. Acta Otolaryngol 116:74–76

84. Koch U, Pau HW (1994) Tubenfunktionsstörungen. In: Naumann HH, Helms J, Herberhold C, Kastenbauer E (eds) Oto-Rhino-Laryngologie in Klinik und Praxis. Thieme, Stuttgart, pp 564–581

85. Kong SK, Lee IW, Goh EK, Park SH (2011) Autologous cartilage injection for the patulous Eustachian tube. Am J Otolaryngol 32:346–348

86. Kujawski OB, Poe DS (2004) Laser Eustachian tuboplasty. Otol Neurotol 25:1–8

87. Kumazawa T, Iwano T, Ushiro K et al (1993) Tubotympanoplasty. Acta Otolaryngol (Suppl) 500:14–17

88. Lapidot A, Kapila A (1967) Experimental construction of a "new" Eustachian tube. Arch Otolaryngol 86:38–44

89. Leuwer R (1996) EMG-Analyse von muskulären Funktionsstörungen der Tuba auditiva. Habilitationsschrift, Hamburg

90. Leuwer R (2004) Acute otitis media/otitis media with effusion in children with cleft palate. In: Alper CM, Bluestone CD, Casselbrant ML, Dohar JE, Mandel EM (eds) Advanced therapy of otitis media. BC Decker, Hamilton, pp 465–467

91. Leuwer R, Henschel M, Sehhati-Leuwer S, Hellner D, Eickhoff W (1999) Ein neuer Aspekt zur Entstehung chronischer Mittelohrerkrankungen bei Patienten mit Gaumenspalte. Laryngo-Rhino-Otol 78:115–119

92. Leuwer R, Koch U (1999) Anatomie und Physiologie der Tuba auditiva – Therapeutische Möglichkeiten bei chronischen Tubenfunktionsstörungen. HNO 47:514–523

93. Leuwer R, Schubert R, Kucinski T, Liebig T, Maier H (2002) The muscular compliance of the auditory tube: a model-based survey. Laryngoscope 112:1791–1795

94. Leuwer R, Schubert R, Wenzel S, Kucinski T, Koch U, Maier H (2003) New aspects of the mechanics of the auditory tube. HNO 51:431–438

95. Lieberum B, Jahnke K (1996) Der goldene Tubendraht zur temporären oder permanenten Implantation. HNO 44:140–142

96. Lim D, Jackson D, Bennett J (1975) Human middle ear corpuscules – a light and electron microscopy study. Laryngoscope 85:1725–1737

97. Lous J (2008) Which children would benefit most from tympanostomy tubes (grommets)? A personal evidence-based review. Int J Pediatr Otorhinolaryngol 72:731–736

98. Lous J, Burton MJ, Felding JU, Ovesen T, Rovers MM, Williamson I (2005) Grommets (ventilation tubes) for hearing loss associated with otitis media with effusion in children. Cochrane Database Syst Rev 25:CD001801

99. Lükens A, DiMartino E, Günther RW, Krombach G (2012) Functional MR imaging of the Eustachian tube in patients with clinically proven dysfunction: correlation with lesions detected on MR-images. Eur Radiol 22:533–538

100. Luntz M, Pitashny R, Sadé J (1991) Cartilage in the bony portion of the Eustachian tube. In: Sadé J (ed) Basic aspects of the Eustachian tube and middle ear diseases. Kugler and Ghedini, Amsterdam, pp 17–22

101. Luschka H (1867) Die Anatomie des menschlichen Kopfes. Verlag der Laupp'schen Buchhandlung, Tübingen

102. Luxford WM, Sheehy JL (1982) Myringotomy and ventilation tubes. A report of 1568 ears. Laryngoscope 92:1293–1297

103. Magnuson B (1978) Tubal closing failure in retraction-type cholesteatoma and adhesive middle-ear lesions. Acta Otolaryngol 86:408–417

104. Magnuson B (1981) On the origin of the high negative pressure in the middle ear space. Am J Otolaryngol 2:1–12

105. Magnuson B (1981) Tubal opening and closing ability in unilateral middle ear disease. Am J Otolaryngol 2:199–209

106. Magnuson B (1983) Eustachian tube pathophysiology. Am J Otolaryngol 4:123–130

107. Magnuson B (1989) The sniff theory. In: Conference on the Eustachian tube and middle ear diseases, Geneva

108. Magnuson B (1991) How to treat tubal malfunction? In: Sadé J (ed) The Eustachian tube and middle ear diseases, basic aspects. Kugler and Ghedini, Amsterdam, pp 289–291

109. Matsune S, Takahashi H, Sando I (1996) Mucosa-associated lymphoid tissue in middle ear and Eustachian tube in children. Int J Pediatr Otorhinolaryngol 34:229–236

110. Matsune S, Sando I, Takahashi H (1992) Elastin at the hinge portion of the Eustachian tube cartilage in specimens from normal subjects and those with cleft palate. Ann Otol Rhinol Laryngol 101:163–167

111. Mayer L (1866) Studien über die Anatomie des Canalis Eustachii. JJ Lentner'sche Buchhandlung, München

112. McCoul ED, Singh A, Anand VK, Tabaee A (2012) Balloon dilation of the Eustachian tube in a cadaver model: technical considerations, learning curve, and potential barriers. Laryngoscope 122:718–723

113. McDonald MH, Hoffman MR, Gentry LR, Jiang JJ (2012) New insights into mechanism of Eustachian tube ventilation based on cine computed tomography images. Eur Arch Otorhinolaryngol 269:1901–1907

114. McGrew BM, Jackson CG, Glasscock ME (2004) Impact of mastoidectomy on simple tympanic membrane perforation repair. Laryngoscope 114:506–511

115. Merchant SN, McKenna MJ, Rosowski JJ (1998) Current status and future challenges of tympanoplasty. Eur Arch Otorhinolaryngol 255:221–228

116. Milewski C (1993) Composite graft tympanoplasty in the treatment of ears with advanced middle ear pathology. Laryngoscope 103:1352–1356
117. Miller JB (1962) Patulous Eustachian tube in pregnancy. West J Surg Obstet Gynecol 70:156–159
118. Miralles R, Gutiérrez C, Zucchino G, Cavada G, Carvajal R, Valenzuela S, Palazzi C (2006) Body position and jaw posture effects on supra- and infrahyoid electromyographic activity in humans. Cranio 24:98–103
119. Mishiro Y, Sakagami M, Takahashi Y (2001) Tympanoplasty with and without mastoidectomy for non-cholesteatomatous chronic otitis media. Eur Arch Otorhinolaryngol 258:13–15
120. Misurya VK (1974) Surgical treatment of the abnormally patulous Eustachian tube. J Laryngol Otol 88:877–883
121. Misurya VK (1975) Tympano-nasopharyngeal shunt operation. A new method of middle ear ventilation. J Laryngol Otol 89:189–197
122. Morita M, Matsunaga T (1988) Effects of an anti-cholinergic on the function of patulous Eustachian tube. Acta Otolaryngol (Suppl) 458:63–66
123. Münker G (1980) The patulous Eustachian tube. In: Münker G, Arnold W (eds) Physiology and pathophysiology of the Eustachian tube and middle ear. Thieme, Stuttgart, pp 113–117
124. Munro KJ, Benton CL, Marchbanks RJ (1999) Sonotubometry findings in children at high-risk from middle ear effusion. Clin Otolaryngol 24(3):223–237
125. Murti K, Stern R, Cantekin EI, Bluestone CD (1980) Sonometric evaluation of the Eustachian tube function using broadband stimuli. Ann Otol Rhinol Laryngol 89(suppl 68):178–184
126. Nguyen LHP, Manoukian JJ, Yoskovitch A, Al Seibeih KH (2004) Adenoidectomy: selection criteria for surgical cases of otitis media. Laryngoscope 114:863–866
127. Nunn DR, Derkay CS, Darrow DH, Magee W, Strasnick B (1995) The effect of very early cleft palate closure on the need for ventilation tubes in the first years of life. Laryngoscope 105:905–908
128. Nuutinen J, Kärjä J, Karjalainen P (1983) Measurement of mucociliary function of the Eustachian tube. Arch Otolaryngol 109:669–672
129. Ockermann T, Reineke U, Upile T, Ebmeyer J, Sudhoff HH (2010) Balloon dilatation eustachian tuboplasty: a clinical study. Laryngoscope 120:1411–1416
130. O'Connor AF, Shea JJ (1981) Autophony and the patulous Eustachian tube. Laryngoscope 91:1427–1435
131. Ogawa S, Satoh I, Tanaka H (1976) Patulous eustachian tube. A new treatment with infusion of absorbable gelatin sponge. Arch Otolaryngol 102(5):276–280
132. Oshima T, Kikuchi T, Hori Y, Kawase T, Kobayashi T (2008) Magnetic resonance imaging of the Eustachian tube cartilage. Acta Otolaryngol 128:510–514
133. Oshima T, Kikuchi T, Kawase T, Kobayashi T (2010) Nasal instillation of physiological saline for patulous Eustachian tube. Acta Otolaryngol 130:550–553
134. Ozturk K, Snyderman CH, Sando I (2011) Do mucosal folds in the Eustachian tube function as microturbinates? Laryngoscope 212:821–824
135. Pahnke J (1991) Beiträge zur klinischen Anatomie der Tuba auditiva. Medizinische Habilitationsschrift, Würzburg
136. Pahnke J (2004) Morphology, function, and clinical aspects of the Eustachian tube. In: Jahnke K (ed) Middle ear surgery. Thieme, Stuttgart, pp 1–22
137. Pahnke J, Hoppe F, Hofmann E, Preisler V (1990) Funktionelle Anatomie des Ostmannschen Fettkörpers. HNO 47:428
138. Park K (2011) Otitis media and tonsils–role of adenoidectomy in the treatment of chronic otitis media with effusion. Adv Otorhinolaryngol 72:160–163
139. Pau HW (2011) Eustachian tube and middle ear mechanics. HNO 59:953–963
140. Pau HW, Sievert U, Just T, Sadé J (2009) Pressure changes in the human middle ear without opening the Eustachian tube. Acta Otolaryngol 128:1182–1186

141. Plate S, Johnsen NJ, Nodskov Pedersen S, Thomsen KA (1979) The frequency of patulous Eustachian tubes in pregnancy. Clin Otolaryngol 4:393–400

142. Plester D (1961) Problems of tympanoplasty. J Laryngol Otol 75:879–884

143. Poe DS (2007) Diagnosis and management of the patulous Eustachian tube. Otol Neurotol 28:668–677

144. Poe DS, Silvola J, Pyykko I (2011) Balloon dilation of the cartilaginous Eustachian tube. Otolaryngol Head Neck Surg 144:563–569

145. Prasad KC, Hegde MC, Prasad SC, Meyappan H (2009) Assessment of Eustachian tube function in tympanoplasty. Otolaryngol Head Neck Surg 140:889–893

146. Proctor B (1967) Embryology and anatomy of the Eustachian tube. Arch Otolaryngol 86:503–514

147. Proctor B (1973) Anatomy of the Eustachian tube. Arch Otolaryngol 97:2–9

148. Pulec JL (1967) Abnormally patent eustachian tubes: treatment with injection of polytetra-fluoroethylene (Teflon) paste. Laryngoscope 77:1543–1554

149. Pulec JL (1980) Diseases of the eustachian tube. In: Paparella MM, Shumrick DA (eds) Otolaryngology. Saunders, Philadelphia/London/Toronto, pp 1402–1421

150. Pulec JL, Hahn FW (1970) The abnormally patulous Eustachian tube. Otolaryngol Clin North Am 3:131–140

151. Pulec JL, Simonton KM (1964) Abnormal patency of the Eustachian tube. Report on 41 cases. Laryngoscope 74:267–271

152. Putz R, Kroyer A (1999) Functional morphology of the pterygoid hamulus. Anal Anat 181:85–88

153. Rajion ZA, Al-Khatib AR, Netherway DJ, Townsend GC, Anderson PJ, McLean NR, Samsudin AR (2012) The nasopharynx in infants with cleft lip and palate. Int J Pediatr Otorhinolaryngol 76:227–234

154. Reiter R, Haase S, Brosch S (2009) Repaired cleft palate and ventilation tubes and their associations with cholesteatoma in children and adults. Cleft Palate Craniofac J 46:598–602

155. Rich AR (1920) A physiological study of the Eustachian tube and its related muscles. Johns Hopkins Hosp Bull 352:206–214

156. Rich AR (1970) A physiological study of the Eustachian tube and its related muscles. Otolaryngol Clin North Am 3:147–162

157. Robinson PJ, Hazell JW (1989) Patulous eustachian tube syndrome: the relationship with sensorineural hearing loss. Treatment by eustachian tube diathermy. J Laryngol Otol 103:739–742

158. Robinson PJ, Lodge S, Jones BM, Walker CC, Grant HR (1992) The effect of palate repair on otitis media with effusion. Plast Reconstr Surg 89:640–645

159. Robison JG, Wilson C, Otteson TD, Chakravorty SS, Mehta DK (2012) Increased eustachian tube dysfunction in infants with obstructive sleep apnea. Laryngoscope 122:1170–1177

160. Rocabado M (1983) Biomechanical relationship of the cranial, cervical, and hyoid regions. J Craniomandibular Pract 1(3):62–66

161. Rüdinger N (1870) Vergleichende Anatomie und Histologie der Ohrtrompete. JJ Lentner'sche Buchhandlung, München

162. Sadé J (2005) Invited commentary to: Van der Avoort et al. (see below). Otol Neurotol 26:543

163. Sadé J, Ar A (1997) Middle ear and auditory tube: middle ear clearance, gas exchange, and pressure regulation. Otolaryngol Head Neck Surg 116(4):499–524

164. Sadé J, Luntz M (1991) Adenoidectomy and otitis media. Ann Otol Rhinol Laryngol 100:226–231

165. Sakakihara J, Honjo I, Fujita A, Kurata K, Takahashi H (1993) Compliance of the patulous Eustachian tube. Ann Otol Rhinol Laryngol 102(2):110–112

166. Sakamoto Y, Akita K (2004) Spatial relationships between masticatory muscles and their innervating nerves in man with special reference to the medial pterygoid muscle and its accessory muscle bundle. Surg Radiol Anat 26:122–127

167. Sakikawa Y, Kobayashi H, Nomura Y (1995) Changes in middle ear pressure in daily life. Laryngoscope 105:1353–1357

168. Sando I, Takahashi H, Aoki H, Matsune S (1993) Mucosal folds in human Eustachian tube: a hypothesis regarding functional localization in the tube. Ann Otol Rhinol Laryngol 102:47–51

169. Sando I, Takahashi H, Matsune S, Aoki H (1994) Localization of function in the Eustachian tube: a hypothesis. Ann Otol Rhinol Laryngol 103:311–314

170. Schliephake H, Hausamen JE (2012) Lippen-Kiefer-Gaumenspalten. In: Hausamen JE, Machtens E, Reuther J, Eufinger H, Kübler A, Schliephake H (eds) Mund-, Kiefer-, Gesichtschirurgie, 4th edn. Springer, Berlin

171. Schrom T, Kläring S, Sedlmaier B (2007) Treatment of chronic tube dysfunction. Use of the tube conductor. HNO 55:871–875

172. Seagle MB, Nackashi JA, Kemker FJ, Marks RG, Williams WN, Frolova LY, Gonchakov GV, Scheslavsky S (1998) Otologic and audiologic status of Russian children with cleft lip and palate. Cleft Palate Craniofac J 35:495–499

173. Seedorf H, Leuwer R, Fenske C, Jüde HD (2002) Das Costen-Syndrom – welche Befunde lassen aus HNO-ärztlicher Sicht die Zusammenarbeit mit einem Zahnarzt sinnvoll erscheinen? Laryngo-Rhino-Otol 81:268–275

174. Sehhati-Chafai-Leuwer S, Wenzel S, Bschorer R, Seedorf H, Kucinski T, Maier H, Leuwer R (2006) Pathophysiology of the Eustachian tube – relevant new aspects for the head and neck surgeon. J Craniomaxillofac Surg 34:351–354

175. Seif S, Dellon AL (1978) Anatomic realtionships between the human levator and tensor veli palatine and the Eustachian tube. Cleft palate J 15:329–336

176. Shimokawa T, Yi SQ, Izumi A, Ru F, Akita K, Sato T, Tanaka S (2004) An anatomical study of the levator veli palatini and superior constrictor with special reference to their nerve supply. Surg Radiol Anat 26:100–105

177. Sheahan P, Miller I, Sheahan JN, Early MJ, Blayney AW (2004) Longterm otological outcome of hamular fracture during palatoplasty. Otolaryngol Head Neck Surg 131: 445–451

178. Sheer FJ, Swarts JD, Ghadiali SN (2010) Finite element analysis of Eustachian tube function in cleft palate infants based on histological reconstructions. Cleft Palate Craniofac J 47:600–610

179. Siedentop KH (1972) Eustachian tube dynamics, size of the mastoid air cell system, and results with tympanoplasty. Otolaryngol Clin North Am 5:33–44

180. Siedentop KH, Hamilton LR, Osenar SB (1972) Predictability of tympanoplasty results. Preoperative Eustachian tube function and size of mastoid air cell system. Arch Otolaryngol 95:146–150

181. Smith TL, DiRuggiero DC, Jones KR (1994) Recovery of Eustachian tube function and hearing outcome in patients with cleft palate. Otolaryngol Head Neck Surg 111:423–429

182. Smith CG, Paradise JL, Sabo DL, Rockette HE, Kurs-Larsky M, Bernard BS, Colborn DK (2006) Tympanometric findings and the probability of middle ear effusion in 3686 infants and young children. Pediatrics 118:1–13

183. Smith W, Yung M (2006) How we do it: laser reduction of peritubal adenoids in selected patients with otitis media with effusion. Clin Otolaryngol 31:69–72

184. Songu M, Aslan A, Unlu HH, Celik O (2009) Neural control of Eustachian tube function. Laryngoscope 119:1198–1202

185. Spindel JH, Lambert PR, Ruth RA (1995) The round window electromagnetic implantable hearing aid approach. Otolaryngol Clin North Am 28:189–205

186. Stangerup SE, Tjernström O, Harcourt J, Klokker M, Stokholm J (1996) Barotitis in children after aviation; prevalence and treatment with Otovent. J Laryngol Otol 110:625–628

187. Stroud MH, Spector GJ, Maisel RH (1974) Patulous Eustachian tube syndrome. Preliminary report of the use of the tensor veli transposition procedure. Arch Otolaryngol 99:419–421

188. Suehs OW (1960) The abnormally open Eustachian tube. Laryngoscope 70:1418

189. Sudhoff H, Brors D, Al-Lawat A et al (2006) Posterior canal wall reconstruction with a composite cartilage titanium mesh graft in canal wall down tympanoplasty and revision surgery for radical cavities. J Laryngol Otol 120(10):832–836

190. Sudhoff H, Schröder S, Reineke U, Lehmann M, Korbmacher D, Ebmeyer J (2013) Therapy of chronic obstructive eustachian tube dysfunction: evolution of applied therapies. HNO 61:477–482

191. Swarts JD, Alper CM, Luntz M, Bluestone CD, Doyle WJ, Ghadiali SN, Poe DS, Takahashi H, Tideholm B (2013) Panel 2: Eustachian tube, middle ear, and mastoid – anatomy, physiology, pathophysiology, and pathogenesis. Otolaryngol Head Neck Surg 148(4 Suppl):E26–E36

192. Takahashi H (2001) The middle ear. The role of ventilation in disease and surgery. Springer, Tokyo

193. Takahashi H, Hasebe S, Sudo M (2004) State of Eustachian tube function in tympanoplasty. In: Alper CM, Bluestone CD, Casselbrant ML (eds) Advanced therapy of otitis media. BC Decker, Hamilton/London

194. Takasaki K, Hirsch BE, Sando I (2000) Histopathologic study of the human Eustachian tube and its surroudings structures following irradiation for carcinoma of the oropharynx. Arch Otolaryngol Head Neck Surg 126:543–546

195. Takasaki K, Sando I, Balaban CD, Miura M (2002) Functional anatomy of the tensor veli palatine muscle and ostmann's fatty tissue. Ann Otol Rhinol Laryngol 111:1045–1049

196. Takasaki K, Takahashi H, Miyamuto I, Yoshida H, Yamamoto-Fukuda T, Enatsu K, Kumagami H (2007) Measurement of angle and length of the Eustachian tube on computed tomography using the multiplanar reconstruction technique. Laryngoscope 117:1251–1254

197. Tasker A, Dettmar PW, Panetti M, Koufman JA, Birchall JP, Pearson JP (2002) Reflux of gastric juice and glue ear in children. Lancet 359:493

198. Tideholm B, Brattmo M, Carlborg B (1999) Middle ear pressure: effect of body position and sleep. Acta Otolaryngol 119(8):880–885

199. Todd NW, Saunders AZ (1991) Patulous eustachian tube: an adult sequel to childhood otitis media. In: Sadé J (ed) The Eustachian tube and middle ear diseases, basic aspects. Kugler and Ghedini, Amsterdam, pp 265–271

200. Tos M (1972) Tympanoplasty in chronic adhesive otitis media. Acta Otolaryngol 73:53–60

201. Tos M (1974) Permanent middle-ear aeration in tympanoplasty. J Otorhinolaryngol Relat Spec 36:170–178

202. Tos M (1979) Middle ear pressure following tympanoplasty for various middle ear diseases. Acta Otolaryngol Suppl 360:148–151

203. van der Avoort SJC, van Heerbeek N, Zielhuis GA, Cremers CWRJ (2005) Sonotubometry: Eustachian tube ventilatory function test: a state-of-the-art review. Otol Neurotol 26:538–543

204. van Heerbeek N, Ingels KJ, Snik AF, Zielhuis GA (2001) Eustachian tube function in children after insertion of ventilation tubes. Ann Otol Rhinol Laryngol 110:1141–1146

205. Virtanen H (1978) Patulous Eustachian tube. Acta Otolaryngol (Stockh) 86:401–407

206. Virtanen H, Palva T (1982) Surgical treatment of patulous Eustachian tube. Arch Otolaryngol 108:735–739

207. Vrabec JT, Deskin RW, Grady JJ (1999) Meta-analysis of pediatric tympanoplasty. Arch Otolaryngol Head Neck Surg 125:530–534

208. Warwick R, Williams PL (1973) Gray's anatomy. Longman, Edinburgh

209. Wehrs RE (1981) Aeration of the middle ear and mastoid in tympanoplasty. Laryngoscope 91:1463–1468

210. Wenzel S (2004) Die Verschlussinsuffizienz der Tuba auditiva – Neue Aspekte zur Pathogenese, Diagnostik und Therapie von Mittelohrprotektionsstörungen. Habilitationsschrift, Hamburg

211. Wimmer E, Toleti B, Berghaus A, Baumann U, Nejedlo I (2010) Impedance audiometry in infants with a cleft palate: the standard 226-Hz probe tone has no predictive value for the middle ear condition. Int J Pediatr Otorhinolaryngol 74:586–590

212. Wullstein HL (1958) The surgical restoration of hearing in chronic otitis media and its audio-logical basis. Ann Otol Rhinol Laryngol 67:952–963
213. Yañez C, Pirrón JA, Mora N (2011) Curvature inversion technique: a novel tuboplastictech-nique for patulous Eustachian tube—a preliminary report. Otolaryngol Head Neck Surg 145:446–451
214. Yoshida H, Kobayashi T, Takasaki K, Takahashi H, Ishimaru H, Morikawa M, Hayashi K (2004) Imaging of the patulous Eustachian tube: high-resolution CT-evaluation with multi-planar reconstruction technique. Acta Otolaryngol 124:918–923
215. Zahnert T, Hüttenbrink KB, Mürbe D et al (2000) Experimental investigations of the use of cartilage in tympanic membrane reconstruction. Am J Otol 21(3):322–328
216. Zöllner F (1942) Anatomie, Physiologie, Pathologie und Klinik der Ohrtrompete und ihre diagnostisch-therapeutischen Beziehungen zu allen Nachbarschafterkrankungen. In: Zange J (ed) Hals-, Nasen-, Ohrenheilkunde der Gegenwart und ihre Grenzgebiete. Springer, Berlin

Index

J.L. Dornhoffer et al., *A Practical Guide to the Eustachian Tube*,   71
DOI 10.1007/978-3-540-78638-2, © Springer-Verlag Berlin Heidelberg 2014